Motor Development in the
Different Types of
Cerebral Palsy

DEDICATION

To our Swiss friend Dr Elspeth Koeng, in acknowledgment of her great pioneer work in the field of early treatment of the child with cerebral palsy

Motor Development in the Different Types of Cerebral Palsy

By
Berta Bobath, *FCSP*
and
Karel Bobath, *MD, FRCPsych, DPM*

Heinemann Physiotherapy

London

First published 1975
Reprinted 1976
Reprinted 1981
Reprinted 1982
Reprinted 1984
Reprinted 1985

ISBN 0 433 03333 9

Printed in Great Britain by
The Whitefriars Press Ltd., London and Tonbridge

Foreword

Dr and Mrs Bobath are rightly famous for their observations on children with cerebral palsy. The treatments they devised and have improved over the last twenty years are based on sound neuro-developmental principles and are outstanding among the welter of eponymous "methods".

In this book they describe motor development in the different types of cerebral palsy. It will be extremely useful to physiotherapists and paediatric neurologists involved in the assessment and care of such children.

We are fortunate in having the views of these two eminent people available to all of us. We are all grateful to them for their contribution to our knowledge and we are grateful to them for this book.

Ronald Mac Keith DM FRCP

formerly Director, Newcomen Clinic, Guy's Hospital, London, SE1 9RT.

Introduction

Great changes take place during a baby's growth and maturation in abnormal as well as in normal motor development. Normal motor development means the gradual unfolding of a child's latent abilities. The baby's early and fairly simple movements change and become more varied and complex. Stage by stage, former achievements are modified, elaborated and adapted to suit finer and more selective movement patterns and skills. This process continues for many years, but the greatest and fastest changes take place in the first 18 months, during which time the most fundamental and important milestones are reached. By this time, the child is able to get up against gravity, walk with some balance and use his hands for manipulation, though still rather clumsily. There are many things he still cannot do, which will develop in the future and change his activities further. Up to about 3 years of age, the improvement in balance and hand skills continues at a fairly quick rate. He learns to walk faster and on a narrower base, to run, to feed himself, to help with dressing and undressing, to play with toys and to speak.

At about the age of 5, he is ready for school. He now has good control of his balance, can jump, play games and can co-ordinate selective and precise movements of his hands for manual skills. He is ready to learn to write. From now on, development slows down and no drastic or quick changes take place, although co-ordination and skills continue to improve during the rest of his school life.

The child with cerebral palsy also develops, but at a slower rate. His development, however, is not only retarded, but follows an abnormal course. In severe cases, that is to say, in children whose whole body is affected, there may be but little change for a long time or development may become arrested altogether at a very early stage. Furthermore, whereas the changes in the development of a normal child's motor patterns are most rapid and significant up to about 5 years of age, changes in the activities of a child with cerebral palsy are slowed down but may continue into adolescence or even adult life. This is especially so in the case of some athetoids and in ataxic children, who remain mobile and do not easily develop contractures and deformities. Indeed, some athetoid children do not acquire walking until they are 14 or 15 years of age.

DEVELOPMENTAL DIAGNOSIS

It is a fact that the diagnosis of cerebral palsy in early infancy — that is to say, in a baby of up to 4, or even 6, months of age — is difficult. In a few babies, the early signs of some deviation from the normal may disappear spontaneously and the children subsequently develop normally though some clumsiness and difficulty with finer selective movements, together with problems of perception may be discovered at school age (Rosenberg and Weller, 1973). Many of the milder cases may have seemed to have been physically normal or fairly normal in early infancy and to have shown only some retardation of development with little progress. These early signs of retarded development may lead to a diagnosis of mental retardation alone, unless there are also obvious signs of physical abnormality. All children with cerebral palsy reach their milestones later than is normal and this regardless of intelligence and degree of involvement. It is so not only in the quadruplegic child, but also in the diplegic and hemiplegic. There may be little change in a child's activities during the first 12 months — in severe cases for 18 months, even — when, in normal circumstances, this is the time of greatest change. Further, added to the delay in maturation, sooner or later, depending on the severity of the individual case, a deviation from normal development takes place, seen in the appearance of abnormal motor activities. These appear when the baby becomes more active, that is, when he tries to sit up, to use his arms and hands, to pull himself to standing, or when he tries to walk in spite of his physical difficulties. Spasticity,

2

athetosis, or ataxia then appear: they become more pronounced in time and the abnormality of the child's postural and movement patterns increasingly obvious. This development and increase of abnormal activity interferes with, and makes impossible, normal motor development. The child therefore tries to function with an inadequate equipment of motor patterns, using the lesser affected or unaffected parts of his body in compensation. Many of the essential and fundamental patterns of motor development, which emerge in a normal child at certain stages of growth, in preparation for future, more complex activity, are missing. The child's development is therefore not only delayed but disordered and disturbed as a result of the lesion.

MILESTONES AND DEVELOPMENT
THE NORMAL CHILD

The milestones of normal child development and the way in which normal children move at various ages are well-known and fairly predictable. Milestones are activities which a normal child reaches at certain chronological stages, artificially isolated and taken out of the context of his all-round development. They are used for testing a child's motor and mental progress and have a value in the detection and diagnosis of motor and mental retardation, particularly in those cases where there are no signs of pathological deviation. Development, however, does not proceed in a linear sequence of separate milestones. At any stage of a child's development, when he reaches a specific milestone, many other, and equally important, abilities are attained which belong to that same stage. The growing baby gains certain basic abilities, such as head and trunk control, arm support and balance, i.e. increasing postural control against gravity. These abilities find expression in a number of related activities and not only in a particular milestone.

Some stages of this development, such as the levels reached at 3, 5, 7 and 9 months of age, described as follows, mark the achievement of certain important abilities, which prepare the child for new and more complex activity and therefore seem of special significance.

3

The 3 months' stage

This is a stage of preparation for midline orientation. Although there is still much flexion in supine, head raising in prone, with forearm support, prepares for increasing extension of trunk and of the lower limbs.

The 5 months' stage

During this stage, further extension and symmetry take place. In prone-lying, the child raises his head well, with extension and abduction of his limbs, supports himself on extended arms and begins to reach out. He pulls himself up from supine against gravity in spite of strong extensor activity in both supine and prone. Also in supine, he pushes his hips up in preparation for extensor activity in later standing and, when sitting supported, he tends to throw himself back. The Landau and parachute reactions are now present, both being part of the child's increasing ability to extend against gravity. Trunk balance in sitting is still lacking. The first equilibrium reactions in prone and supine appear.

The 7–8 months' level

The child now achieves rotation within the body axis (the body righting reaction on the body modifying the total rotation of the early neck righting reaction). The baby rolls over from prone to supine and from supine to prone. He will need such rotation for creeping and getting up from prone to sitting. At 8 months, he can balance in sitting without arm support, and use his arms sideways when losing balance. Balance reactions in sitting are active. He starts to pull himself up to standing, but cannot as yet get on hands and knees.

The 9–10 months' stage

At this stage, the child begins to crawl on all fours, on hands and feet, or alternately with one knee and one foot on the ground. He pivots and gets about in sitting, and can also walk along furniture or when held by both hands. He still needs balance in standing and cannot therefore walk unaided or does so, initially, on a wide base with widely abducted legs.

It can thus be seen that the great changes that take place in the normal child, and the increasing development of a variety of spontaneous activities, are based on, and made possible by, the gradual increase in postural control against gravity. As the righting reactions develop and become perfected, around the sixth, or seventh month, they are modified and incorporated into the equilibrium reactions. The developing parachute reactions of the arms are equally important. Together with this development, we see a change in the motor patterns of the limbs from the flexion-adduction of the newborn, through flexion-abduction, towards extension-abduction. From the seventh month onwards, the extension-abduction patterns of the limbs become combined with rotation of the trunk. This is a necessary prerequisite of normal equilibrium reactions. The following short summary of related activities belonging to certain stages of normal development may be of interest:

3-4 months

The flexion-adduction pattern of the limbs in earliest infancy has now changed to flexion-abduction.

The development of head control and of forearm support and midline orientation are shown in the following ways:

Prone Head up to midline; extension sufficient for forearm support; midline orientation.

Supine Head in midline; hands engage; arms flexed; legs flexed-abducted.

Pulled to sitting Head kept in line with trunk, still some initial head lag.

Sitting Trunk has to be supported, head fairly steady when trunk is moved.

5 months

Symmetry. The beginning of extension-abduction of limbs and the Landau reaction, shown as follows:

Prone Further extension; swimming on floor, legs abducted-extended, lifted off the support. Arms either forward, almost extended and used for support, or retracted at shoulders and flexed, with hands off the support. Towards the end of this period, the child supports himself on one forearm and reaches out for a toy with the other. Turns from prone to supine. Landau begins.

Supine Strong extension of shoulders and back; elbows flexed; legs flexed-abducted. However, arms can be brought forward and hands can be brought to midline. Rolls to either side. At 5 months, can arch his back and lift his hips to make a "bridge", thus practising extension. Begins to lift his head.

Pulled to sitting Head comes forward. He assists in sitting up. Legs are lifted off support in flexion-abduction.

Sitting Very insecure, no balance or arm support. Arms retracted at shoulders with flexed elbows. Tends to throw himself backwards or falls backwards.

Standing If supported, begins to take his weight, still on adducted legs.

6 months

Strong extension-abduction of limbs. Strong righting reactions. Landau stronger. Head control in supine and prone good. These find expression in:

Prone Full extension and support on fully extended arms. Reaching out with one hand for toy while supporting himself with the other. Legs extended and abducted.

Supine Reaching forward when mother picks him up. Lifting legs and playing with feet. Foot to mouth. Rolling to prone. (Extension-abduction allows for rotation — body righting reaction on body begins.)

Pulled to sitting Raising legs with extension, lifting head off support, pulling himself to sitting.

Sitting Arm support forward but still tends to fall

backwards. Sitting unsupported, briefly, no trunk balance yet.

Standing   Bouncing, weight carried on more abducted legs.

7 to 8 Months

Beginning of trunk rotation. Trunk control and sitting balance develop, Landau very strong. Parachute reaction forward and sideways present. These find expression in:

Prone   Going from prone to sitting. Pivoting in prone. Pushing himself backwards or pulling himself forwards with arms. Creeping and getting up to sitting over one side.

Supine   Dislike of this position (strong righting reactions). Rolling over or sitting up.

Sitting   Sitting unsupported for one minute. Leaning forward with arm support (7 months). Sitting steadily with good balance, and recovering balance with arm support sideways (8 months).

Standing   Pulling himself to standing holding onto furnitures, but not yet crawling on hands and knees.

8-10 months

Beginning of locomotion. Landau very strong. Sitting balance perfect. Beginning of arm support backwards. These find expression in:

Prone   Crawling on hands and knees, on hands and feet, or on one foot and one knee.

Sitting   Pivoting, good balance without arm support. Going from crawling to sitting and back to crawling.

Standing   Legs widely abducted. Walking, holding onto furniture or held by both hands.

To sum up, this short survey gives examples of related activities at various stages of a child's motor development. It shows how certain basic features, such as better control against gravity, head control, rotation, arm support and equilibrium reactions, enable a child to develop his overt activities simultaneously in various directions. It also shows that progress is not linear and that there is a great overlap of abilities. This summary is concerned with motor development only: the more specialised aspects of development, i.e. of visio-motor control, prehension and manipulation, speech and language development have been described in great detail by other writers (Sheridan, Griffiths, Gesell and Illingworth). They are, however, obviously and closely related to the development of general motor ability.

THE COMPETITION OF MOTOR PATTERNS
IN NORMAL CHILD DEVELOPMENT

As mentioned before, different activities at specific stages of normal development interact with each other. They may reinforce each other, or may compete with each other for a short while. This idea of "competition of motor patterns", put forward by Milani (1964), is a most valuable one. He says: "The dynamic process of motor structuration in the early stages of infantile development appears to be essentially an interweaving of various patterns which appear and disappear, and interfere with each other in their mutual interacting and modulating influence with an orderly integration in the developmental process."

When a child tries to do something new, which is still difficult for him, he will "practise" the new pattern with great perseverance. He will concentrate on it for many days, or even weeks. Former activities may be discontinued for a time, or they may deteriorate in performance due to the effort of doing something new and difficult. Once the new pattern has become established and easy, the earlier ones are taken up again and become part of the one newly achieved. Examples of this are the "primary responses", such as the stepping response, the crossed extension, primary standing and automatic walking, as described by Andre Thomas and Dargassies (1960), which deteriorate or disappear between 2 and 6 months of age. MacKeith (1964), however, has shown thatautomatic walking can for a longer time still be elicited by raising the baby's head. The baby no longer takes weight on his legs as in primary standing and the well co-ordinated movements of automatic walking deteriorate. At 5 months, if made to stand, the child will not take weight on his legs but will draw them up in flexion. When automatic walking is attempted, his legs drag along, he remains on his toes and does not dorsiflex his feet as he did before.

Between 3 and 8 months of age, strong extension of the trunk and arms against gravity develop from the head downwards, and with it the child's upper limbs become more active than his legs. Extension at this time is excessive and is a dominant pattern which seems to interfere with the former well co-ordinated movements of his legs. When, later on, the child starts to take weight on his legs again, they are at first extended and adducted, his feet are plantiflexed, and his toes flexed in grasp response. His feet may be "so disorientated that he may stand on the dorsum of his feet" (Thomas and Dargassies, 1960).

The dominance of one pattern over others can also be seen in babies who are nursed mainly lying in prone. They may gain extension of head and trunk in prone very early, but head control from supine is then achieved later than is normal. Other babies, who are nursed in sitting and supine-lying, may lift their heads from supine very early. They show good head control when pulled to sitting from supine, but they cannot push themselves up on their arms from prone-lying until much later than is usual.

Some children never crawl on all fours but get about the floor in sitting. They have been called "shufflers" by Robson (1970, 1973). He suggests that the cause of this is a phase of non-persistent hypotonia. He says "shuffling is preceded by a phase of hypotonia, dislike of prone-lying and hip flexion posture in vertical suspension which makes the infant appear to be reluctant to weight-bear on his lower limbs. . . . The presence of hypotonia causes them eventually to find a way of moving about in a sitting position 'shuffling'."

If hypotonia were the sole reason for the baby's inability to get on hands and knees and to crawl, it would seem logical to assume that it would also interfere with his ability to get up to sitting and to shuffle. As the child dislikes the prone position, it would seem to be more likely that he was not put into this position, but nursed in sitting for a long time. A child will soon prefer sitting to prone lying, as he can see people and his surroundings more easily than when lying on the floor in

9

prone. He can also use his hands for play with greater ease. There may also have been insufficient floor space to allow the baby to creep in prone, as most children do, prior to crawling and walking. The pattern of sitting with flexed hips would then become dominant and compete with, and delay, extension of the hips for weight-bearing in standing. The same would apply to support on extended arms. This might account for the fact that "shufflers" are late walkers.

Another good example of the "competition of patterns" and the disturbing influence of the dominance of one pattern over another, can be seen in children who, at about 18 months, return to the bilateral use of their hands for a while, as described by Illingworth (1960), after previously having used their hands unilaterally or bilaterally. This temporary regression to bilaterality—i.e. to a 4 to 7 months' level—may be due to a child walking on a wide base with arms in a pattern of symmetrical abduction, in order to maintain balance. This symmetrical extension-abduction pattern of upper and lower limbs is dominant at this stage, and seems to interfere with the already established former patterns of rotation of the trunk and reciprocal movements of the arms which had developed when sitting safely.

MILESTONES OF DEVELOPMENT AND TREATMENT IN CEREBRAL PALSY

The milestones and abnormal motor patterns of the child with cerebral palsy, as in the case of normal babies, are also fairly predictable, but they are different in the various types of cerebral palsy and not so well known.

The comparison of normal with abnormal development in terms of milestones, for the purpose of a diagnosis, and especially as a guide for the treatment of cerebral palsy, is inadequate and unsatisfactory. As has been said, the main cause of the child's delay in reaching certain milestones is not only retardation but pathology, that is, his neurological deficit. This shows itself in various types of abnormal postural tone — flaccidity, spasticity, rigidity, or the fluctuating tone of the athetoid group — and in abnormal

10

patterns of posture and movement closely associated with it. Development in cerebral palsy should be assessed in terms of the modification of patterns of co-ordination, in terms of the interplay of developing normal and abnormal postural reactions, rather than by milestones. This will not only help towards a better understanding of the reasons for developmental delay or failure to reach certain milestones, but will also allow for a proper assessment of the nature of the child's handicap and be an adequate guide for treatment. Assessment in terms of milestones has far too often led to a diagnosis of mental retardation.

THE CONCEPT OF MOTOR DEVELOPMENT AS A SUCCESSION OF MILESTONES

This concept also has a danger in that it leads to a rigid and dogmatic way of concentrating treatment on obtaining a few activities, one after another. This can be very dangerous, as it will reinforce one or two patterns of activity for too long a time, to the exclusion of others of equal importance, belonging to the same stage of the child's development. It disregards the concept of "competition of patterns" and may lead to a permanent deterioration and even loss of former activities. The long-term reinforcement of one or two patterns, such as creeping or crawling, and the disregard of patterns functionally and developmentally related, will also interfere with the achievement of new activities.

In treating a child with cerebral palsy, one should not try to perfect one activity before going on to the next. This may take a very long time, and the patterns of movement thus developed will become dominant over any other. As we have noted before, the normal baby does not perfect one activity before going on to the next; for instance, he achieves sitting balance only at a time when he can already stand; he can crawl on hands and knees at a time when he is already beginning to pull himself up to standing and can even walk, holding on to a support; he begins to walk when balance reactions in standing develop.

In cerebral palsy, with an abnormal postural tone and co-ordination, the exclusive practice and reinforcement in treatment of one or two activities, performed in abnormal ways over a lengthy period of time will either prevent progress or make any new and more difficult activity merely be a modification of the original abnormal patterns. This, in the spastic child, would lead to the development of contractures and deformities. For instance, a spastic child who has reached the stage of sitting and crawling, but who cannot stand or walk, activities which belong to the same stage of development, is in danger of developing flexor deformities of hips and knees and this pattern of flexion will become dominant in the course of time. The athetoid child and the ataxic child, who have a great variety of abnormal postural and movement patterns, are not in such danger of developing deformities, as no one pattern can become dominant. This does not, however, apply to the dystonic type of athetoid or to cases of mixed spasticity and athetosis. These children may also develop contractures in time, though usually not so quickly as we see it happen in the pure spastics.

DIAGNOSIS AND PROGNOSIS

As mentioned before, the diagnosis of cerebral palsy is very difficult in babies under 4 months of age or even at 6 months, if they are only mildly affected. This is because the very young infant does not usually show much abnormality. The signs will be predominantly those of retardation of motor development and the retention of primitive reactions. A differential diagnosis, that is, a diagnosis of the *type* of cerebral palsy, is even more difficult to arrive at with any certainty during the first 6 months, or even later. The differential diagnosis of the so-called "floppy" baby is especially difficult as many of them later become athetoid or ataxic or they may be found to be suffering from conditions other than cerebral palsy. Children who are diagnosed early as spastic quadruplegias may turn out later on to be

12

athetoids, or cases of mixed spasticity and athetosis. The extent of the involvement of a baby's body may also be difficult to forecast. Frequently, babies are diagnosed as monoplegias with only one arm affected but later turn out to be hemiplegias. A child diagnosed as a hemiplegia in early infancy may later turn out to be a quadruplegia, the more involved side having shown pathology earlier. Spastic paraplegias may show some involvement of the arms and hands much later on, often not until they are at school. Spastic diplegias quite frequently are diagnosed late, that is, not before a delay in sitting up is noticed, which may not be until the baby is 9 months of age. In milder cases, the diagnosis may not be made before 18 months, when the child should be walking.

As the cerebral palsied child becomes more active, abnormal postures and movements develop and will change as the child adapts them to functional activities. These changes follow fairly predictable lines but are still different in the various types of cerebral palsy, and in spastic quadruplegias and diplegias, hemiplegias and athetoids.

A knowledge of these changes in the child's condition is of great importance. It may help the doctor to discover the earliest signs of abnormality, to supervise and guide treatment, and to prevent some, or most, of the predictable changes for the worse. Unfortunately, prognosis remains uncertain and results of treatment unpredictable until the child has reached a fairly stable stage of development. This may not be before the child is 5 years old, or even later, especially in some children with ataxia or athetosis.

Babies who are diagnosed as slight cases and therefore likely to respond quickly to early treatment, may turn out to be more severely affected than was expected and need treatment for a long time. These are often the intelligent children, who try too hard and get on to their feet and use their hands for self-help too soon, the effort unfortunately reinforcing their abnormal patterns. On the other hand, there are babies who seem to be quite severely affected but who, against all expectations, give good and fairly quick treatment results. These factors make prognosis at an early age uncertain.

In spite of these uncertainties care should be taken not to miss the best time when treatment can influence and improve the quality of co-ordination in the child's developing activities, and the child helped, thereby, to mature in the most normal way possible.

In all these cases there is a delay in milestones. In many premature babies and in those with a stormy birth history, undue delay in reaching milestones is thought to be normal and pathology is not suspected. Diagnosis and treatment are then postponed.

In a few children, early abnormal signs may disappear spontaneously and the children develop normally, though in some children, as mentioned before, difficulties with fine selective movements and skills as well as perception problems may be discovered at school age (Doran Benyon, 1968; Rosenberg & Weller, 1973). The differentiation between slight deviations from the normal and mild signs of abnormality, is sometimes extremely difficult. In such cases, especially when the babies are under 4 months of age, postponement of treatment is justifiable but only if a careful watch is kept and frequent checks made on their further development. Should treatment be given, a child may respond very well and may be normal at about 12 months of age; but one may doubt whether this result and the claims which are sometimes made to have "cured" a child, or "prevented the development of cerebral palsy" are due to the effect of treatment. There is no harm in treating a baby under 3 or 4 months of age, but one should not claim success as a result of treatment nor include such children in any statistics. On the whole, we think it is better to keep the child under careful observation, and to start treatment only if the early signs do not disappear or if they become more obvious.

The critical period seems to be at 4 months of age. Signs of abnormality may then become more obvious, and diagnosis easier as the child grows older. The physical condition then deteriorates, compared with the apparent normality seen earlier, when diagnosis was difficult and the delay in milestones was thought possibly to be due to mental retardation.*

* *See* Appendix, p. 101.

THE DIFFERENTIATION BETWEEN PRIMITIVE
AND ABNORMAL PATTERNS

It is difficult to draw a clear dividing line between slight abnormal signs of brain damage and the primitive normal movement patterns seen in babies under 3 or 4 months of age, but an attempt to do so could be useful for diagnosis and for therapy.

One might define "primitive patterns" as belonging to the very early stages of normal child development, roughly from birth to 3 or 4 months of age. "Abnormal motor patterns" might be defined as those not seen at any stage of a normal full term baby's development.

The difficulty of very early diagnosis arises from the fact that both types of motor behaviour are found in all cases of cerebral palsy with a consequent retardation or arrest of motor development. In very young infants and in the slightly affected older children, the *primitive* patterns predominate, while in the older and more severely affected children the *abnormal* patterns are more pronounced.

Primitive normal movement patterns can indicate pathology, in the following ways:

1. If they are tested one by one without relating them to other activities belonging to the same stage of development, some of which may be missing. There may be a wide scatter of movement patterns belonging to different stages of development. This happens in diplegic and hemiplegic children who achieve activities of later stages with the lesser or unaffected parts of their body, while early stages are still missing in the affected parts.
2. If they are combined with abnormal postural tone, such as hypertonus, hypotonus or fluctuating tone.
3. If seemingly normal and primitive patterns are stereotyped and limited, in contrast to the great variability of movements found in the normal child.

   The following are some examples:

   Grasp of hands *only* with flexed pronated arm and with flexion of head and trunk.

15

Opening of hands *only* when the head is thrown backwards and no isolated movements of the fingers occur.

Forearms *always* pronated and never supinated. Obligatory asymmetrical tonic neck reflexes when the head is turned to one side, even if this happens before the end of the 16th week.

Retraction of the shoulders with flexed elbows *without* being able to get hand to mouth or both hands together in midline.

The head *always* turned to one side.

The elbows *never* extended except when head is turned to one side or as part of the Moro reaction.

Grasping with one hand *only* and not with the other.

Head control forwards when pulled to sitting *but no* head lifting in prone.

Ability to turn from prone to supine *but not* from supine to sides.

Ability to turn from supine to side-lying *but not* from side-lying to supine.

Kicking with one leg only *but no* reciprocal kicking.

Flexion of legs *only* with abduction and simultaneous flexion at all joints, *but no* independent movements of ankles or knees.

Plantiflexion of toes *without* being able to dorsiflex them.

Supination of ankles *without* being able to pronate them.

Mouth *always* open, lips never close.

Extension of elbows *only* with internal rotation at shoulder.

Thrusting backwards of head and trunk when sitting *without* being able to bring the head forward when pulled to sit.

Definite abnormal signs such as internal rotation of the legs, asymmetries of the trunk and neck, adduction of legs and plantiflexion of ankles (as well as others) have not been mentioned here as they are well known and they present no diagnostic problem.

DEVELOPMENT OF SPASTICITY

Only a few children are spastic or rigid at birth. They are usually the very severely affected spastic quadruplegics. Some of the children who are rigid to begin with, may become "filoppy" later on. In most cases, spasticity develops gradually as the child matures and starts to react to his development.

The children who are stiff very early on, show opisthotonus, a stiff spine and extended legs in supine. Their arms are retracted at the shoulders and flexed at the elbows.

The same children show *flexor* spasticity of the neck, trunk and hips in prone-lying and are unable to lift the head. If extensor spasticity is very strong in supine, some children may also extend their hips and knees in prone. They may be able to lift the head in prone due to tonic extension being strong even in prone. This pattern shows a combination of stiff extension of the adducted legs with flexion and adduction of the arms. If one tries to flex one knee, or both, the tonic extension suddenly changes to a total flexor pattern and the head can no longer be lifted.

Children who do not show spasticity or rigidity early on, have fairly normal postural tone during the first 4 months of life. Hypertonus develops slowly and tonic reflex activity increases, which is in contrast to the normal child, where the occasional influence of the asymmetrical tonic reflexes disappears around the fourth month. In the normal child *extensor* activity in prone develops from the head downwards until, at about 5 months, his hips and knees are fully extended in prone. In the child with cerebral palsy, however, *flexor* spasticity of trunk and arms in prone prevent him from lifting his head and extending spine and hips.

Unless propped up in sitting, the cerebral palsied child remains lying on his back. This position increases neck and shoulder retraction and extensor spasticity of the trunk becomes stronger. Gradually his legs extend with adduction, internal rotation and plantiflexion of ankles and toes. When the child is made to stand supported, e.g. when being dressed, extensor spasticity of ankles and toes increases still further.

When sitting supported, his head bends forward and

downward and his back is flexed. Thus, the total pattern of flexor spasticity becomes superimposed on the original extensor pattern, a mixture of two total abnormal patterns. We then see flexion of the spine combined with retraction of the flexed arms, and semi-flexion of the hips and legs with adduction and internal rotation. When the child lifts his head, he extends his trunk and hips, his knees extend, the adduction increases and his legs may cross. If not supported, he falls on his back.

When standing supported, a similar mixed pattern of tonic flexor and extensor activity is seen. With his head bent forward, the child's shoulders are protracted and his arms flexed while his legs are stiffly extended and adducted. His hips are somewhat flexed and, with his head flexed forward, his ankles are dorsiflexed and he keeps his heels down. When he raises his head, his spine and hips extend, his shoulders retract, adduction and internal rotation of his hips increase, and he stands on his toes and is in danger of falling backwards. Later on, in order not to fall backwards and when trying to walk, he will avoid lifting his head, thus keeping his hips and knees in some flexion, and he will stand on his toes in order to prevent a collapse into a total flexor pattern.

Development of intermittent spasms

Intermittent spasms, sometimes called "tensions", occur mainly in children who are "floppy" early on. The arms and legs are usually flexed and abducted at rest. These children often turn out to be athetoid, ataxic, or mixed conditions later on. On stimulation, and when they are excited, sudden extensor thrusts of the whole body occur with rigid extension of neck, spine and hips. Asymmetrical tonic neck reflexes can be seen in conjunction with extensor thrusts. The knees and feet are usually less affected by these spasms, and adduction, with internal rotation at the hips, occurs only later when the child is made to stand up or when he sits supported and tries to use his hands. As long as the legs are mainly flexed and abducted — often excessively abducted in flexion — the feet are dorsiflexed and pronated. Supination of the ankles develops gradually with extension and adduction. However,

18

the tendency towards adduction and crossing of the legs can often be seen when lifting the child up under the axillae.

In contrast to the spastic children who combine flexor with extensor patterns, we see sudden alternations between total flexion and total extension. This change from rigid extension to a sudden collapse in flexion, is a great problem for postural control and fixation in sitting and standing. Usually the extensor spasms become stronger in time when the child tries to maintain a posture against gravity.

STAGES OF ABNORMAL MOTOR DEVELOPMENT

A foreknowledge of the abnormal ways which a child with cerebral palsy will use to achieve some functional skills, gives the therapist the means to intercept such development at the right time, i.e. at the first signs of abnormal patterns before they become established and habitual. It also gives the doctor a better chance to make an early diagnosis and may help towards an earlier prognosis.

By frequently observing a child's motor development, i.e. the quality of his motor patterns, the doctor and the therapist have common ground for co-operation in the planning of treatment, and for the necessary subsequent changes in the treatment plan, thus keeping the treatment in step with the child's changing condition and activities.

The changes of motor patterns which will be discussed later have been divided into three stages for each type of patient. This has been done in order to indicate the outstanding changes which take place as the child develops new activities, i.e. when he learns and tries to function in spite of his handicap. These "stages of abnormal development" should not be regarded as "milestones" to be seen at certain chronological ages. It may take years for a child to progress from one stage to the next, and many children may never get beyond the first, or second stage. Much depends on the severity of the individual child's involvement and on his intelligence. Generally, one might say that the spastic child's progress along these stages will have reached its peak *before* he is 6 or 8 years of age, while in the athetoid and ataxic child progress from stage to stage may continue until the age of 15 or even later.

The changes of motor patterns are fairly typical and have been observed by the authors in many children during more than 30 years' work with the cerebral palsied, though deviations from these patterns can and will occur in the individual case.

Before describing the natural history of the different types of this condition in some detail, it is necessary to define their classification:

Diplegia The whole body is involved but the legs more than the arms. The distribution of spasticity is usually more or less symmetrical. The children usually have good head control and moderate to slight involvement of the upper limbs. Speech is usually unaffected. All diplegic children belong to the spastic group. Strabismus is present in a number of children.

Quadruplegia The whole body is affected. In athetoid quadruplegias the upper limbs and the trunk are usually more affected than the lower limbs. In spastic quadruplegias and in some mixed cases the lower limbs may be involved to the same extent as the arms. There is a considerable difference in the involvement of the two sides of the child's body resulting in pronounced asymmetry of posture and movement. Head control is poor and there is usually impairment of speech and eye co-ordination.

Many spastic children and all patients of the athetoid group belong in this category as do children with ataxia, flaccidity or rigidity. Many cases are of a mixed character. They may show spasticity with athetosis or athetosis with ataxia. Babies may gradually develop rigidity, athetosis or ataxia after having been hypotonic initially, or signs of athetosis when initially they showed only spasticity.

Hemiplegia One side of the body only is involved. The children are usually of the spastic type, but a few may develop some distal athetosis later on. True hemi-athetosis is very rarely seen.

Monoplegia One arm only, or, less frequently, only one leg is involved. They are very rare and usually turn out later to be hemiplegias.

20

Paraplegia In Cerebral Palsy true paraplegias are also very rare. Very few children show no involvement "above the waist" as seen in spinal injuries. They usually turn out to be diplegias with mild involvement of arms and hands, sometimes only of one arm.

Common features of the different types

Because of the typical patterns of spasticity, we find similar patterns of posture and movement in spastic diplegias and spastic quadruplegias. It is therefore not always easy to differentiate a spastic diplegia from a spastic quadruplegia, especially when the upper limbs are only slightly less affected than the lower limbs, as happens in some diplegias. Mixed cases of athetoid quadruplegia with spasticity may show some similarities with spastic quadruplegia as they combine features of spasticity with athetosis. However, if athetosis as well as spasticity is present, the children are more mobile than those with pure spasticity.

There are, therefore, similarities and overlap of symptomatology. For this reason, some repetition in the description of patterns of motor development of the different types of children cannot be avoided.

STAGES OF ABNORMAL DEVELOPMENT

Spastic diplegia

Many of these babies are premature and their slow development is thought to be due to this. Their milestones are delayed but postural tone is fairly normal early on. The physiological excess of flexor tone, seen in very young normal babies, may remain unaltered for many months. Although later than normal, head control develops and the child's arms and hands seem to be unaffected. He can get his hands together in midline and to his mouth and he develops midline orientation of his head. His legs show little spasticity initially; they are flexed and abducted, though full passive abduction may be somewhat resisted. For these reasons,

21

diagnosis is not usually made before about 9 months of age when the child does not sit up by himself and has no balance when made to sit. Some mildly affected children may not be diagnosed until 18 months or even 2 years of age, when they pull themselves up to stand and start walking on their toes. Then they usually show an asymmetrical pattern of standing and walking, one foot on the toes with little weight on that leg, the other foot heel down but with hyper-extension of the knee and flexion of that hip.

First stage. Supine, prone, rolling, creeping and sitting supported

Supine When lying on their backs the diplegic babies may move their legs feebly in semi-flexion; one leg, usually the right one, abducts and flexes more than the other. This asymmetrical "kicking" leads to adduction and internal rotation of the other leg, usually the left, and may be the first sign of the development of a subluxation of that hip (Figs 1). Gradually extension of the legs becomes stronger, combined with increased adduction of both legs and even crossing of the legs. To begin with, this is done with external rotation at the hips, as can be observed in normal babies up to about 4 months of age who extend their legs with some adduction and may even cross their feet occasionally. However, in spastic children internal rotation at the hips occurs gradually as part of extension and adduction. At first, the ankles may still be dorsiflexed but later, when extensor spasticity becomes stronger, they plantiflex and supinate.

Prone When lying face downwards, reciprocal creeping movements of the legs can be seen early on, much like in a normal baby, but again — as in supine — with more flexion and abduction of one leg. While in supine, the legs are still mostly flexed, in prone they extend stiffly and adduct when the baby starts to lift his head, and even more so when he starts to push himself up on his forearms. In normal development the legs are flexed and abducted at this stage.

Whether in prone or supine, there are no independent movements of the ankles or of the knees, which we see very early on in normal babies. Normal babies move their feet up

22

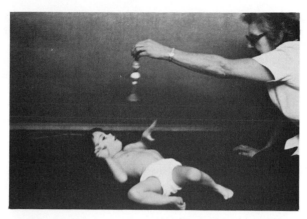

Fig. 1a Spastic diplegia: Retraction of left shoulder prevents the arm from reaching forward. Abduction and flexion of right leg causes adduction and internal rotation of left leg.

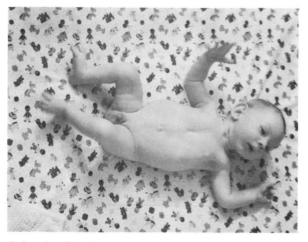

Fig. 1b Spastic diplegia: Abduction and flexion of right leg causes adduction and internal rotation of left leg.

and down and in and out regardless of whether their legs are flexed or extended. They also move their knees independently of hip extension or flexion. The spastic child, however, can only use a total pattern of simultaneous flexion at all joints with abduction at the hip, alternating with extension at all joints with adduction and internal rotation.

Rolling and creeping   Most diplegic children learn to roll from supine to prone and vice versa. They initiate rolling from the head and use their arms while the legs are passive and held stiffly extended and adducted. There is no rotation between pelvis and shoulders (Fig. 2).

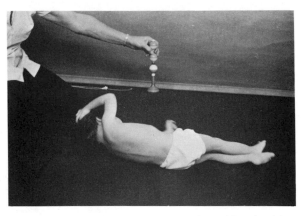

Fig. 2 Spastic diplegia: Rolling supine to prone. Started from head, legs stiff. No rotation within the body axis.

When diplegic children are able to lift their heads in prone and get onto their forearms, they start to get about on the floor. They pull themselves forward with both arms flexed and cannot reach out forwards by lifting and extending their arms reciprocally. The legs are passive and dragged behind (Fig. 3). Some children may be able to push themselves up on to extended arms but they cannot push themselves backwards as normal children do. Neither can they pivot around as they lack rotation of the trunk and abduction of arms and legs. The normal reciprocal creeping movements are missing due to lack of rotation of shoulder-girdle and pelvis. The normal baby may also pull himself along by his arms but he moves his legs reciprocally and he has many other ways of progressing on the floor in prone, such as

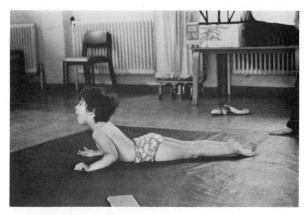

Fig. 3 Spastic diplegia: Pulling herself forward along floor with flexed arms. Legs stiffly extended and passive.

pivoting, pushing himself backwards and "swimming" with reciprocal movements of arms and legs

Gradually, the children's legs become stiff, as the effort of using arms and hands without being able to move their legs produces associated reactions and with it an increase of extensor and adductor spasticity in the legs. When creeping

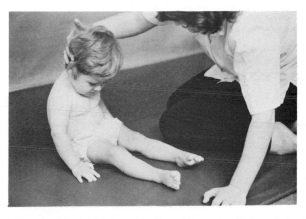

Fig. 4 Spastic diplegia. Made to sit. Round back, insufficient hip-flexion, legs adducted and stiff, feet plantiflexed.

on the floor, some children bend and abduct only one leg, usually the right one, with the head turned to the right side. This asymmetrical pattern will — as mentioned before — increase adduction, internal rotation and extension of the left leg and torsion of the pelvis.

Sitting When made to sit, there is no balance of the trunk. The legs adduct and turn inwards, often more left than right (Fig. 4). The ankles as well as the toes are plantiflexed.

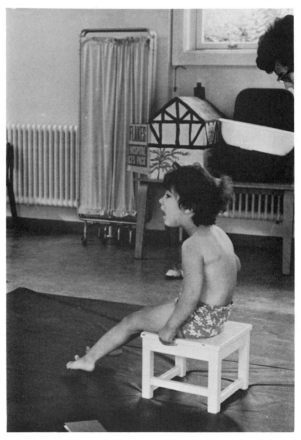

Fig. 5 Spastic deplegia: Sitting on stool. Round back insufficient hip flexion, adducted legs. Note also chin pokes forward.

Unlike the normal child, they cannot sit with their legs extended and abducted (long sitting). The sitting base is therefore narrow, the back very round to compensate for the insufficient flexion at the hips, and the head is flexed or, if the child looks up, the chin is poked forward (Fig. 5). The children tend to extend their hips and to fall backwards when looking up suddenly. The use of arms and hands for support develops late, especially sideways and backwards. In many children, flexion forwards of spine and shoulder girdle prevents this, and support backwards may not become possible at all.

When pulled up from supine to sitting, the legs extend stiffly and adduct, with internal rotation and plantiflexed ankles. The hips resist full flexion (Fig. 6). Head control and also grasp may be good or fairly good and the children may be able to assist sitting up by using their arms.

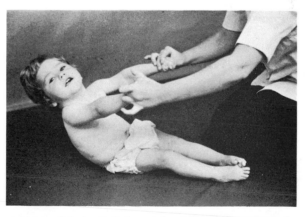

Fig. 6 Spastic diplegia: Pulled to sitting. Note: Hips resist flexion with compensatory kyphosis. Legs stiff, adducted internally rotated, feet plantiflexed.

When starting to sit

There are no balance reactions of the legs and pelvis against falling over to one side. There is also insufficient flexion and abduction at the hips to bring the trunk forwards

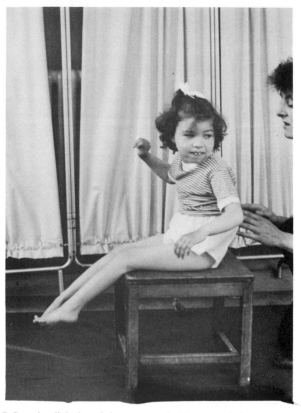

Fig. 7 Spastic diplegia: sitting on stool. Note: no balance. Excessive flexion of spine; compensation for insufficient flexion of hips.

against falling backwards. The child sits on his sacrum and brings his body forward by excessive flexion of his spine (Kyphosis) (Fig. 7). Gradually, support on the arms becomes possible forwards and sideways, but balance of the trunk without arm support remains impossible. Therefore, unsupported sitting is very insecure, and the simultaneous use of both hands for play difficult or impossible. Many children therefore use only one hand for play while supporting themselves with the other. The child cannot lift

28

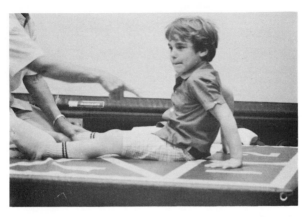

Fig. 8 Spastic diplegia. Arm support backwards. Note child's difficulty. Right elbow flexed.

his arms and extend them to reach out for an object without being in danger of falling backwards or sideways. Reaching upwards while looking up is impossible, often so even if only one arm is used to reach up and the other used for support. There is too much flexion of the spine to get full extension of his arms and he is afraid of falling backwards if he extends his spine. He cannot sit and play on the floor, but if he is made to sit on a chair with a table in front he feels safe as he has no need to balance. He can then use both hands, though some children may still need one hand for support on the table.

Protective extension of the arms (the parachute reaction) is now present forwards and sideways, but always better and more reliable towards one side. Arm support backwards for protection against falling back (normally present at 10 to 12 months) is only possible in a few children with very good arms and hands (Fig. 8).

Second stage. Kneeling, crawling to standing up

The child now wants to get up from the floor but he cannot sit up unaided. Instead of continuing to pull himself along the floor with his flexed arms, he now gets up on to his knees. A

29

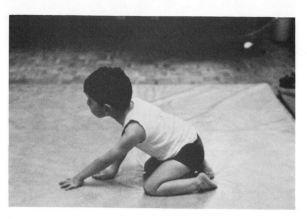

Fig. 9 Spastic diplegia: Pushing himself backwards on to his feet to kneel-sitting.

few children who can support themselves on their extended arms in prone do this by pushing themselves backwards on to their knees (Fig. 9). The legs are passive and adducted. Other children remain on their forearms and pull their legs up under the abdomen until they are on their knees. They then lift the head, extend their arms, put their hands down on the floor, and sit back between their feet (Fig. 10). The legs are adducted and internally rotated at the hips. In this position the children feel safe and can use their hands for play. However, if this position is maintained for long periods of the day, the tendency to internal rotation and adduction will become reinforced and make balance in standing and walking difficult or impossible later on. The normal child uses this position for play at times, but has many other ways of playing when on the floor, such as sitting and squatting. For the diplegic child it is the only way. The posture of the feet is usually asymmetrical, one foot — often the right — is dorsiflexed and pronated while the other is plantiflexed and supinated. If they are also involved, the arms, like the legs, are adducted and internally rotated, the hands often fisted.

At first, most children get about the floor on their seat, or between their feet. They "bunny hop". Later, they learn to get on to their hands and knees and to crawl with small

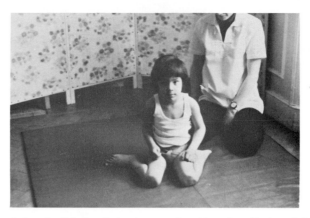

Fig. 10 Spastic diplegia: Sitting between feet. Note: Dorsiflexion of right ankle and plantiflexion of left ankle.

reciprocal movements. The legs remain in semiflexion, the knees remain adducted and the legs internally rotated. Both legs remain in some flexion when crawling, while normally one leg extends when the child moves forward over the weightbearing flexed leg. Though the ankles resist passive dorsiflexion when the legs are extended, they are dorsiflexed when crawling as part of the total flexor patterns (Fig. 11).

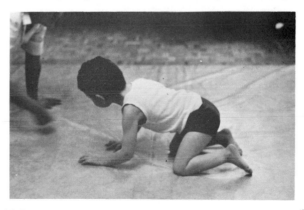

Fig. 11 Spastic diplegia: Crawling in total flexion. Note: Dorsiflexion also of ankles.

31

When on hands and knees, the children cannot seat themselves to one side of their knees (side-sitting) because of lack of rotation of the trunk between pelvis and thorax (Fig. 12). Lack of trunk balance makes it difficult or impossible to play in side-sitting or in long sitting, i.e. with their legs in front as normal children do. At this stage the children cannot stand or walk. Therefore, they sit on a chair or on the floor between their feet most of the time. The exclusive use of flexion of the legs over long periods of time produces flexor contractures at hips and knees.

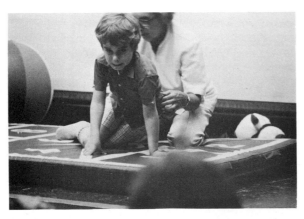

Fig. 12 Spastic diplegia: Side-sitting is difficult.

Standing up Next, the child tries to get on to his feet. From four-foot kneeling he gets up on to his knees, using a chair to hold on. However, he cannot extend his hips fully because his knees are flexed due to the total flexor pattern. Some children extend the hips and bring the pelvis forward but with a lordosis because of flexor spasticity at the hips. The child cannot shift his weight on to one leg in order to bring the other forward to half-kneeling so that he can stand up. He cannot take weight on one extended hip and lift the other leg, bending it at hip and knee, without bending both hips. Therefore, he pulls himself up with his arms straight on to his toes and then moves his feet forwards towards the chair (Fig.

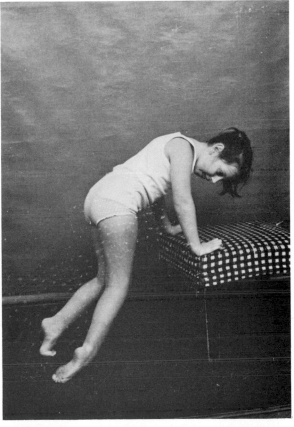

Fig. 13 Spastic diplegia: Standing up child goes on to her toes.

13). Often a child can then only put one heel down to the floor, usually the right one, but only by rotating his pelvis backwards on that side, and with flexion of that hip. The other foot remains on its toes; the leg is internally rotated and does not take weight (Fig. 14). This pattern is a continuation of the asymmetry shown by the child in sitting and when pulling himself along the floor in prone. The rotation of the pelvis with pronounced internal rotation of usually, the left

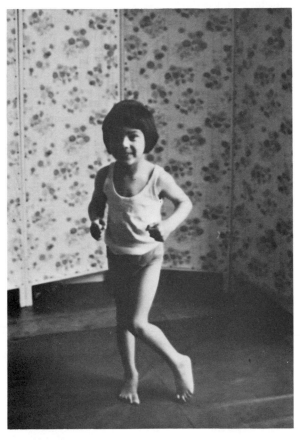

Fig. 14 Spastic diplegia. Standing: Right heel down, left leg adducted and internally rotated, foot on toes. No weight-bearing on left leg.

leg further reinforces the danger of subluxation or dislocation of that hip, especially if walking is done later on in the same asymmetrical pattern as standing.

Third stage. Standing and walking

The child now starts to walk, holding on to furniture or held by one or both hands. Many children walk as mentioned

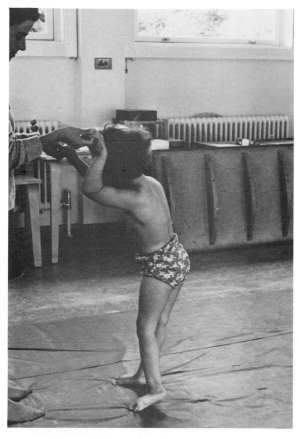

Fig. 15 Spastic diplegia. Helped to walk. Right heel down with flexion of hip. Excessive flexion of trunk and of left arm.

above, that is, with one foot flat on the ground, the other on its toes (Fig. 15). The children cannot move their legs freely to step forwards, sideways or backwards, movements which are needed not only for walking in different directions but even more so for balance. Neither can they shift their weight well over to one foot and balance on it long enough to free the other for making a step (Fig. 16). They stand with their legs stiffly extended and adducted. If they want to walk, they

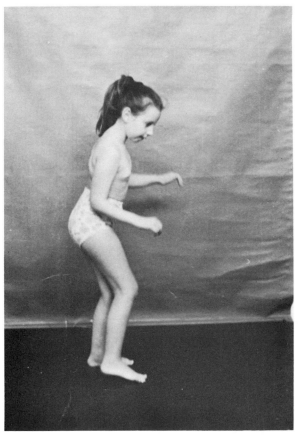

Fig. 16 Spastic diplegia. Walking difficult as child cannot step forward.

need some flexion at hips and knees to give their legs some mobility. Therefore, they start walking with both hips and knees in some degree of flexion, adduction and internal rotation. The weight is then taken on the medial border of the feet which results in a valgus deformity of their feet. As the child cannot take a step while standing safely on the other leg, he moves further forward by bending his trunk over his hips. His legs then follow, toes down first, to prevent him

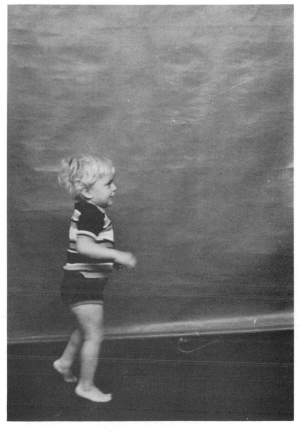

Fig. 17 Spastic diplegia. Walking on his toes.

falling forwards. Even a normal person, walking in this way by moving his body forwards over flexed hips, would be unable to put his heels down first. A gradual tightening of the tendo-achilles will be the unavoidable result of this pattern of walking.

The standing and walking base in the diplegic child is narrow, which makes balance difficult or impossible. Once the child starts walking in this way he cannot stand still but

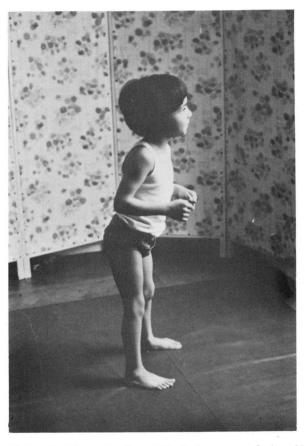

Fig. 18 Spastic diplegia. Standing with heels down causes flexion of hips.

continues to fall from one leg on to the other. He can only stop walking by holding on to a support. The normal child starts standing and walking on a very wide base to get his balance. He first walks sideways along furniture with wide abduction of his legs before he walks forwards. The diplegic child cannot abduct his legs, he cannot walk sideways and has no standing balance without support.

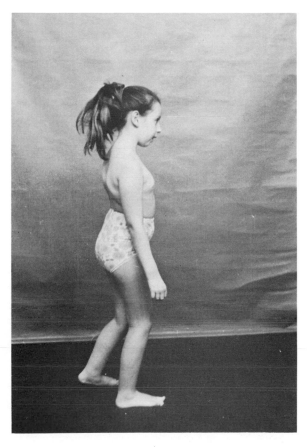

Fig. 19 Spastic diplegia: Standing with a lordosis to compensate for hip flexion.

If spasticity of the legs is slight and the upper limbs and trunk near normal, the child may learn to balance and walk unaided though on a small base and up on his toes (Fig. 17). Other children, mainly those who have a strong tendency to flexion at hips and knees, learn to put their heels down although valgus or "rocker feet" develop through standing and walking with adducted and internally rotated hips and a tight heelcord. Some children may learn to stand

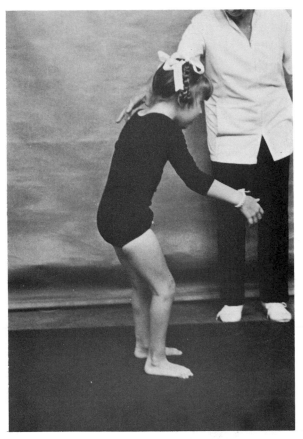

Fig. 20 Spastic diplegia: Lack of balance in standing. Falling backwards in spite of hip flexion.

unsupported as long as their feet are parallel (Fig. 18), but they cannot stand and balance with one foot in front of the other — in step position — which is a necessary part of walking. Many children develop a compensatory lordosis in standing in order to keep head and trunk upright in spite of hip flexion (Fig. 19). There is also an additional danger of developing scoliosis, if — as is often the case — control of

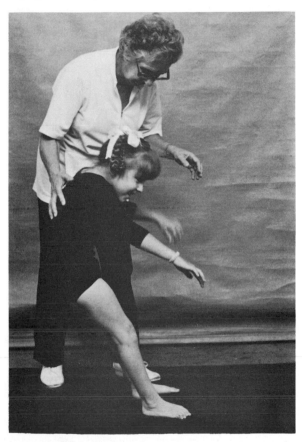

Fig. 21 Spastic diplegia. Weight transferred backwards. Note: Absence of normal dorsiflexion of ankles and toes due to extensor spasticity which pushes child backward.

one hip, usually the left one, is deficient and the child walks with the trunk side-flexed on that side.

All diplegic children tend to fall backwards even if they bend forward at the hips (Fig. 20). They have no balance reactions of the ankles and toes against falling backwards. Instead of the normal dorsiflexion of feet and toes when the body weight is transferred backwards, the balls of their feet press against the ground, the toes plantiflex and push the children back (Fig. 21). Flexion forward at the hips with adduction and internal rotation of the legs will increase in time as the children get older and heavier. The use of walkers and elbow crutches, by perpetuating adduction of the arms and downward pressure from the shoulders, contribute to and reinforce the pattern of flexion of the lower limbs.

A few slightly affected children can abduct their legs and put their heels down when making their first unaided steps. They may start walking fairly normally, much like a normal toddler, but only as long as they walk slowly. There is little spasticity at that stage and balance is possible because of a wide base. However, they soon start to walk faster which increases spasticity. The walking base then becomes narrower, they go up on to their toes, lean forwards at the hips and lose balance in standing and walking.

HEMIPLEGIA

Hemiplegia is often recognised quite early, in fact much earlier than diplegia, because of the obvious asymmetry of the child's postures and movements. A few children are already referred for treatment at 5 months of age. More often, however, they are diagnosed at 8 or 9 months of age or later, when it is noticed that they cannot sit up and when they reach and grasp only with one hand. Some asymmetry of posture is still normal up to about 4 months of age and a diagnosis is therefore difficult unless the hemiplegia is of a severe degree. Furthermore, initially the baby is often referred for treatment with a diagnosis of monoplegia because of constant fisting of the affected hand, while the involved leg appears to be normal.

First stage. Supine, prone, rolling and sitting

Early on, when the hemiplegic child lies on his back, both legs are flexed and abducted, much as they are in normal babies. Though the affected hand is more often fisted than the normal one, at this stage it may still open at times. The baby reaches out for toys with the sound arm and hand only. Retraction of the shoulder with flexed elbows can be seen in normal babies but they can also move their arms and hands for reaching out forwards and they can bring their hands forward to suck their fingers. In the hemiplegic baby, however, the affected arm remains retracted and flexed, or may extend stiffly by his side if his face is turned towards it. He cannot reach forward for toys and he may not be able to get his hands together above his chest nor to put his affected hand to his mouth. As long as he does not yet use his sound hand for play he does not look predominantly towards the sound side. His posture, therefore, is more symmetrical at this early age than later on, when he uses his sound hand exclusively and looks away from the affected side. He does not roll over towards the sound side as he cannot use the affected arm and leg to initiate and perform this movement. Shoulder retraction and the inability to bring the affected arm forward prevents it. Rolling to the side and, later on, to prone is done with the sound side over the affected one.

The hemiplegic child dislikes being in prone as he can support himself on one arm only and cannot reach out and play with the affected one. In this position, the affected arm remains flexed and he has difficulty in moving it out from under his chest.

When wanting to get about on the floor, but not yet able to get up to sitting, some children start to creep in prone. Their face is then turned away from the affected side. They move the sound arm and leg only and drag the affected limbs; they are passive, the leg extended and stiff with internal rotation.

When the child is made to sit, the affected leg remains flexed and abducted, while the normal one extends at the knee (Figs 22a, b). There are no independent movements of knee, ankle and toes. However, when held up to stand, the affected leg, which was flexed and abducted in sitting, now

43

extends and may take weight, while the sound leg may still be drawn up in flexion, such as is seen in both legs in normal babies before they stand (Fig. 23).

Hemiplegic children are late in sitting up and have balance problems, falling easily towards the affected side. Sitting up by themselves from supine or prone is very late. Usually, they get up to sitting from supine by using the sound arm to push themselves up. The effort of doing this on the sound side produces associated reactions with flexion and pronation of the affected arm (Fig. 24). Sitting up from prone-lying, which is earlier in the normal baby than sitting up from supine, is more difficult for the hemiplegic child. He may learn to do this later on, but again only on the sound side, using the sound arm for pushing himself up. Many children miss this important stage of development altogether. They prefer to turn over onto their backs and then sit up. They also do not get onto their hands and knees to sit up nor do they crawl on hands and knees.

When sitting, most of the weight is on the sound hip. The child tends to fall towards the affected side and cannot support himself with the affected arm (Fig. 25). He likes side-sitting only on the sound side, with his weight on the hip of that side. In this position, he gets about the floor on his seat, pushing with the sound arm and pulling himself along with

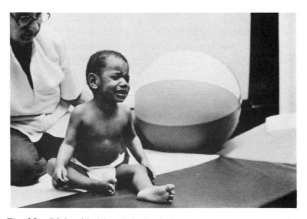

Fig. 22a Right-sided hemiplegia sitting. Note: Right leg flexed.

the sound leg. The affected side is dragged behind and pulled along by the sound one.

From now onwards, flexion and pronation of the affected arm, with retraction of the shoulder and fisting of the hand, become more frequent and are reinforced by associated reactions. The former ability to extend the elbow becomes more and more difficult, or impossible. His interest is focused on the activities of his sound hand and he therefore keeps his head turned towards that side. Gradually he neglects and

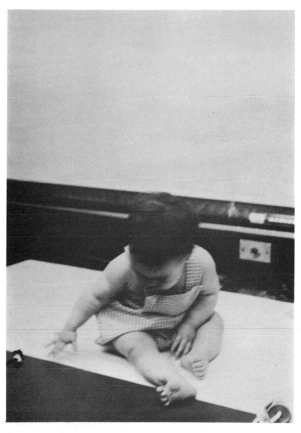

Fig. 22b. Left-sided hemiplegia sitting. Note: Left leg flexed; toes clawing.

45

soon disregards the affected side altogether. Sensory deficits, often present in the arm and hand, contribute to the disregard and even to the complete rejection of the affected arm. Many children hate to be touched on that arm and hand, dislike to look at the hand, and dislike it even more when made to touch the mouth with the affected hand.

Hemiplegic children completely miss the normal bilateral stage of using both hands together in midline and of

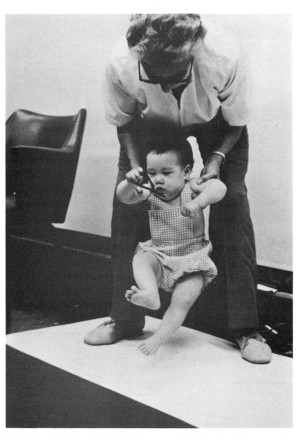

Fig. 23. Left-sided hemiplegia held up vertically to stand. Note: Now left leg extends and adducts, foot plantiflexed and supinated.

transferring objects from one hand to the other. It is interesting that the Moro reaction can be elicited on the affected arm still, and persists for much longer than is normal.

The flexor pattern of the arm is always combined with lateral flexion of the neck and trunk on the affected side.

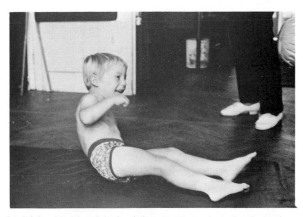

Fig. 24 Right-sided hemiplegia sitting up. Note: Associated reactions with flexion and pronation of right arm with effort.

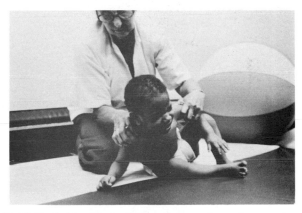

Fig. 25 Right-sided hemiplegia: Sitting. Absence of parachute reaction and support of right arm. Child falls over to the right.

There is resistance to passive flexion of the neck towards the sound side, to extension of the affected side of the trunk and to raising the extended arm. This spastic flexion of the trunk pulls the shoulder-girdle downwards and the pelvis upwards, with apparent shortening of the whole of the involved side and leg.

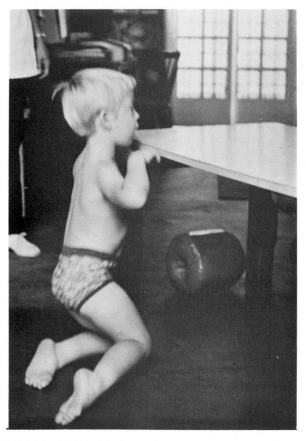

Fig. 26a Right sided hemiplegia standing up. Note: Uses sound hand only. Associated reactions on right arm with strong flexion and pronation of right arm and hand.

Second stage. Standing up and standing

The child now pulls himself up to stand, using the sound hand only. Firstly, he gets onto kneel-standing, then, usually, puts the affected foot forward to half-kneeling as he cannot take weight on the affected flexed knee while keeping his hip

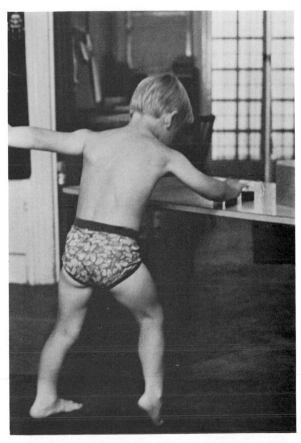

Fig. 26b Right-sided hemiplegia: Standing up. Note: Right foot high on tiptoes. No weight on right leg. When use of normal arm and hand is prevented, there are no associated reactions on right arm. He can extend it to reach for a toy.

extended. When halfway up to standing on the affected leg, he quickly moves the sound foot forward to take the weight standing up (Figs 26a, b, c).

When standing, all weight is on the sound leg, the affected one held abducted. The foot is slightly behind the normal one, because of the backward rotation of the pelvis on the affected side. The shoulder — like the pelvis — is also pulled

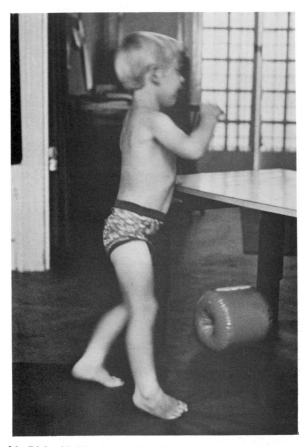

Fig. 26c Right-sided hemiplegia: Standing up. Note: Extensor spasticity of right leg and foot. The foot is on its toes and supinated. There is no weight on it.

backward and the arm flexed (Fig. 27). At this stage, the heel of the affected leg is still on the ground and the leg seems to be more "weak" than spastic, though the toes "claw" the ground and are stiff. When one tries to make the child take weight on the affected leg, by lifting the other passively, he collapses on it.

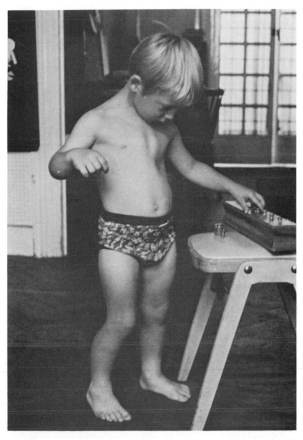

Fig. 27 Right-sided hemiplegia: Standing and playing with left hand. Note: Right shoulder and pelvis pulled backwards. The whole of the body weight on left leg. Associated reactions on right arm with increased flexion while using left arm.

Third stage. Walking

The child now walks held by one hand. Unfortunately, the mother is apt to hold the child by his sound hand. This reinforces his tendency to bring his sound side forward and to leave the affected one behind. He usually keeps the affected leg extended at the knee, abducts it and drags it

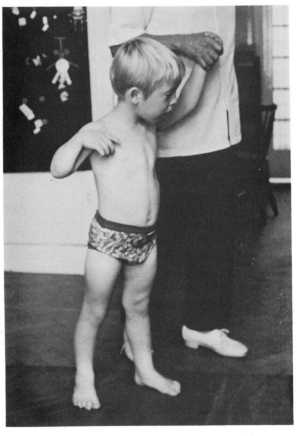

Fig. 28 Right-sided hemiplegia: Walking held by left hand. Note: Right leg extended and abducted. Shoulder and pelvis retracted. Strong associated reactions on arm.

behind the sound side. His shoulder retracts, the elbow is flexed and the hand fisted (Fig. 28). Walking unaided is late, because of balance problems. He is afraid of falling to the affected side as he cannot use his arm for protective support if he should fall. He has no "parachute reactions" and no ability to take weight on that arm. If he should fall to that side, which happens when he is suddenly pushed by other children at play, he falls on the side of his face and bruises his arm and leg. To protect himself, therefore, he orientates himself completely towards the sound side and avoids taking full weight on the affected leg. Balance rections of the affected hip and leg therefore cannot develop. In many untreated children, there is a considerable difference in length and circumference of the leg, which is probably due to this lack of weight-bearing and to the lack of proprioceptive stimulation promoting growth. This impairment of growth in the arm and hand is more pronounced even with early treatment because the use of the upper limb is more limited and often impossible in many children.

In the early stages of unaided walking, he may still put his heel on the ground with the leg held abducted and externally rotated. The child may be able to squat on the ground and

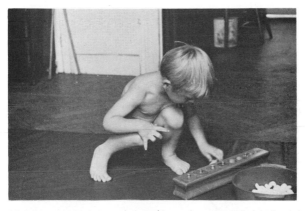

Fig. 29 Right-sided hemiplegia squatting. Note: The whole body weight is on the left leg. The right foot is on tip-toe. The leg placed to one side. The right arm shows flexion with pronation of forearm and wrist.

53

play like a normal child in this position but all his weight is on the sound leg, the other one abducted and placed to one side (Fig. 29). The child will then stand up from squatting, with all his weight on the sound leg. He then starts to walk, using the same pattern of abduction of the affected leg, as he did in squatting. Later, when he walks faster and needs a narrower base, his walking pattern changes. If spasticity is slight, he bends his hip and knee and lifts his leg too high up

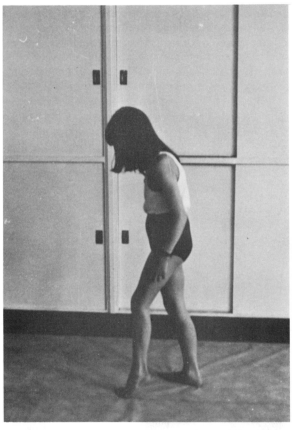

Fig. 30a Left-sided hemiplegia: Making a step forward. Putting toes down first.

when making a step. This brings his toes down first, the heel following. Putting his toes down first produces extensor spasticity and stiffens the ankle due to an exaggerated positive supporting reaction (Fig. 30a). He can, therefore, only put his heel down by bending his hip, and this makes him hyper-extend the knee (Fig. 30b). As part of the increasing extensor spasticity, supination of the ankle develops, with progressive tightening of the heel cord. If

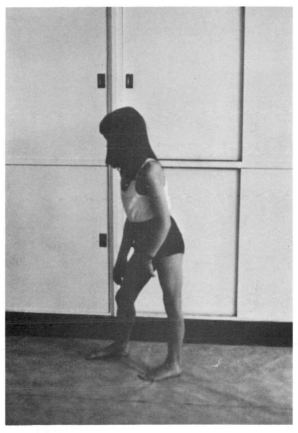

Fig. 30b Left-sided hemiplegia. When putting down heel the hip flexes with hyper-extension of knee.

extensor spasticity becomes still stronger and the heelcord tighter, he is unable to put his heel down any longer and he remains on his toes. The knee then no longer hyper-extends, but remains semi-flexed.

The difficulty and effort involved in learning to balance and to walk unaided and faster increases the flexion and pronation of the hemiplegic arm and hand still more. When the child runs, the whole arm pulls up and abducts at the

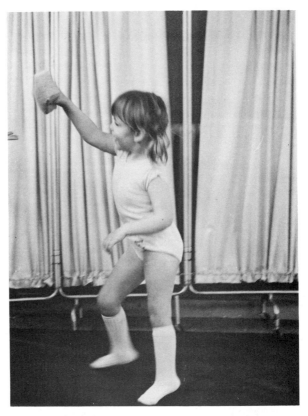

Fig. 31 Left-sided hemiplegia reaching for toy with sound arm. Note: Retraction of the whole left side. The left leg is stiff in extension the ankle plantiflexed, the child on her toes. The left arm shows increased flexion (associated reactions).

shoulder. Many children, who could still use the affected arm and hand at the earlier stages, for instance when playing with large toys which needed the use of both hands, have by now developed such strong flexor spasticity in the arm that they cannot open the hand any longer or reach for and grasp objects. When encouraged to use the affected hand, they can only open their fingers to grasp, with extreme flexion of the wrist. The hand is pronated and deviated towards the ulnar side. Using the hand in this way reinforces the already existing pronation and flexion still further, and results both in flexor and pronator contractures of wrist and elbow. When the child approaches a toy he walks — as mentioned before — leading with the sound side and he reaches out and forward with the sound arm. This pattern perpetuates the backward rotation of his pelvis and the retraction of his shoulder-girdle on the affected side (Fig. 31).

ATHETOID QUADRUPLEGIA

Many athetoid children present the picture of a "floppy infant", to begin with. Postural tone against gravity is very low. The child is passive and placid and there is little spontaneous movement. There are great feeding problems and often abnormal respiration. Bronchitis and broncho-pneumonia are frequent occurrences as the child may be too weak even to cough. His mouth is loosely open, his grasp weak or non-existent. His head is turned to one preferred side, often the right. His hands are open with flexed wrists and elbows. There is usually pronounced asymmetry of the trunk. In some children, the Galant reflex may be present and strong for a long time, even for years, and sometimes can be elicited on only one side (Fig. 32). Head control is usually absent altogether when pulling the child to sit, in sitting supported, and in prone-lying. The child dislikes prone-lying as he cannot lift his head and look around. Sometimes, in this position, breathing is difficult for him, with the face down, and his inability to turn it to one side.

His legs often show an exaggerated primitive flexor pattern; they are excessively abducted (Figs 33a, b). The feet are dorsiflexed and pronated. It is possible to bend the toes to his shin for many months or even for years; this can be done with normal babies but only for a few weeks. Extension of the legs is weak and incomplete. The legs are rather passive, though one leg, usually the right, may move more than the left. There may be weak reciprocal but no simultaneous kicking. With extension of the legs there is some adduction but no internal rotation at the hips. The typical athetoid movements with their abnormal co-ordination do not develop

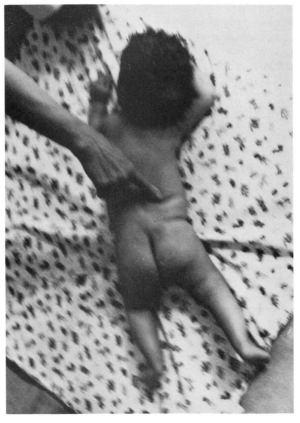

Fig. 32. Athetoid quadruplegia. Galant reflex.

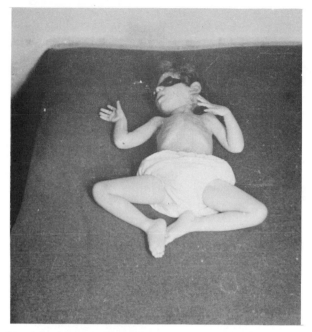

Fig. 33a Athetoid quadruplegia. Primitive flexor pattern with excessive abduction of legs in supine.

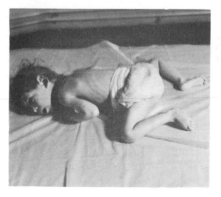

Fig. 33b Athetoid quadruplegia. Primitive flexor pattern with excessive abduction of legs in prone.

until later, often not until 18 months or even 2 or 3 years of age. They seem to develop when the child becomes more active and tries with effort to respond to external stimulation.

First stage. Supine, prone and pulled to sitting

As the baby becomes more active and reacts to his environment, he becomes excited and this shows itself in sudden strong extension of his whole body. He pushes his head and shoulders backward when lying on his back or when supported in sitting. These intermittent extensor spasms were called "dystonic attacks" by Ingram (1959) (Fig. 34). With increasing extension in supine, neck and

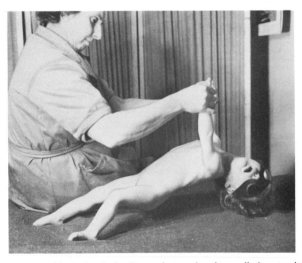

Fig. 34 Athetoid quadruplegia. Dystonic attack, when pulled up to sitting.

shoulder retraction become stronger and the first signs of asymmetrical tonic neck reflexes occur. The child's head is now more or less permanently turned to one side, and many children have difficulty in turning it to the other side, for instance, as when made to follow an object with their eyes. The athetoid child's head is hardly ever in midline. In the early stages, the asymmetrical tonic neck reflex usually affects only the arms while the legs are still mostly flexed and abducted (Fig. 35). He misses the important developmental stage of midline orientation and symmetry with bilateral use of his hands. He cannot move his arms forward and engage his hands or get them to his mouth and suck his fingers. He cannot reach out with his arms to grasp a toy either. When he extends his neck and shoulder-girdle, he tends to open his mouth excessively wide. Later on, we often find that he subluxates the mandible, has difficulty in closing his jaw and lips and dribbles.

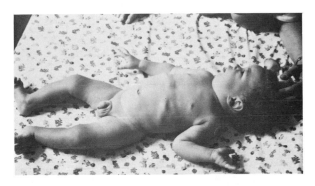

Fig. 35 Athetoid quadruplegia. Asymmetrical tonic neck reflex with head turned to right.

When pulled to sitting, his head not only lags but even pulls backwards due to neck retraction. He cannot, therefore, assist with his arms when pulled to sitting. For many years he is unable to lift his head from supine. Later on, he may learn to assist with his arms when pulled to sitting, using hip flexion to sit up, but with the head still pulling backwards.

If, as is often the case with athetoid children, the legs are less affected than the trunk and upper limbs, he may be able to put his feet onto the support and push his hips up making a "bridge". This activity, which he enjoys as the only one at his disposal, further increases neck and shoulder retraction. Often, the only way of getting about on the floor, is by pushing himself backwards with his legs, an activity which is never seen in normal children. He cannot roll over from supine to prone and, when placed into prone, he cannot lift his head, support himself on his forearms or creep on his tummy. He dislikes being in this position.

Though his legs are still predominantly flexed and abducted, the increasing extensor activity of head and trunk in supine results in more frequent and stronger extension of his legs, which now becomes combined with adduction and

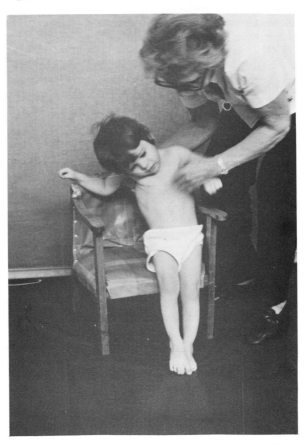

Fig. 36 Athetoid quadruplegia. Made to stand. Extension of legs with adduction. Note: Flexion of right side of trunk and hip due to lateral flexion of neck.

internal rotation. His feet now start to show the typical athetoid pattern of supination with dorsiflexion, instead of the former pronation. He now kicks with one or the other leg and sometimes reciprocally, but simultaneous kicking never develops, as it does in normal babies at about 4 months, when they reach the symmetrical stage of trunk and limbs. If his legs are as much involved as the arms and trunk, which is the case in children who show mixed athetosis with spasticity and also in the "dystonic" child, extension of the legs occurs with strong adduction, internal rotation and crossing (Fig. 36). However, with flexed legs, abduction remains fairly normal for a long time. This is in contrast to the adductor spasticity of spastic children, where some degree of adductor resistance is present when their legs are flexed, though usually it is not as strong as with extended legs.

When made to sit, the athetoid child either falls forward, collapsing at the hips, or, if supported, he tends to push himself backwards. He also tends to fall to one side, usually to the more affected side.

Second stage. Sitting, kneeling, rolling

The child soon wants to move and the effort produces involuntary movements and intermittent spasms of the limbs. Grimacing of the face can also be seen now when he tries to communicate but cannot yet speak. He may now become very excitable and frustrated as he tries to do things without succeeding. He cannot properly co-ordinate, time or direct his movements. He cannot maintain any posture against gravity. Any effort, especially any extension of his head and body is associated with excessive opening of his mouth. He is now in constant motion of body and limbs, especially of hands and feet. He only relaxes and becomes still in sleep, although even then some of the severely dystonic children do not relax.

He cannot sit unsupported and, when made to sit in a chair, he cannot keep his feet on the ground (Fig. 37). If he tries to sit upright, his feet pull up due to excessive flexion at the hips, or his hips and knees extend and he falls backwards

63

against the back of the chair; his hips then slide forward and his legs adduct and often cross (Figs 38a, b). In both situations, he cannot keep his feet on the ground to steady and balance his trunk. As arm support against falling sideways is usually impossible, he cannot keep his hands down on the support even if helped to place them there. Excessive total extension may give way to a complete collapse in flexion forwards, if his hips are held flexed, as by

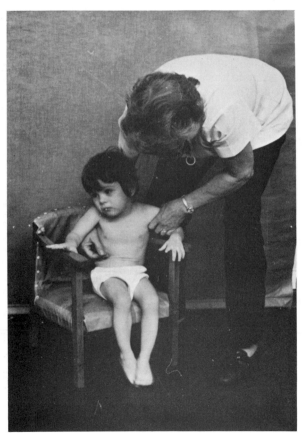

Fig. 37 Athetoid quadruplegia. Child cannot sit unsupported and keep his feet on the ground.

strapping him to the seat of the chair (Figs 39a, b). The asymmetrical posture of his trunk and lack of midline orientation of head and arms result in a scoliosis of the spine and sometimes in subluxation or dislocation of one hip (Fig. 40).

He cannot use his arms for support sideways, forwards or backwards and is unable to reach forward for grasp (Fig. 41). He may try to get one arm forward but can do so only

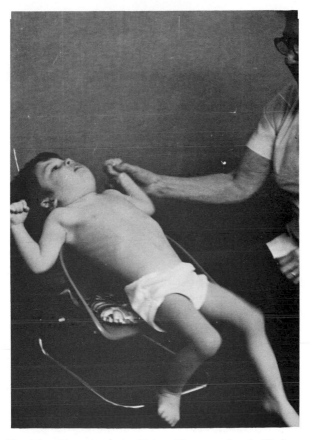

Fig. 38a Athetoid quadruplegia. Sitting: Hips extend and slide forwards and child falls back.

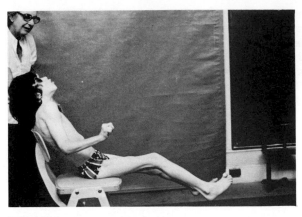

Fig. 38b Athetoid quadruplegia. Sitting: Trying to sit upright and falling backwards. Legs extend and and adduct.

with a rigidly extended elbow and fisted hand, the other arm pulling backwards in either flexion or extension (Fig. 42). If he tries to use one hand in front for play, he tends to fall over to the opposite side. The trunk is unstable as well as asymmetrical. He is unable to move his head independently, his trunk following every movement of his head. When trying to look up or to lift his arms, he will fall backwards; if he looks to one side, he falls to that side and, when looking down, he falls forwards.

Though he cannot yet sit unsupported, he learns to roll over from supine to prone, usually, however, only over one side, using his less affected side. He overcomes the retraction of neck and shoulders by initiating this rolling with the movements of his legs and pelvis, while shoulders and arms follow (Fig. 43). This is in contrast to the child with spastic diplegia, who initiates rolling over with his head and arms, while the legs follow passively. In the prone position, the strong extension of neck and trunk may help the child to lift his head, but he can only do this to one side and not in midline. He cannot hold his head up for any length of time.

When he wants to get up from prone-lying on the floor, he pulls his knees under his abdomen, using a total flexor pattern with his head bent down. He then sits back between his feet, lifts his head and trunk and puts his extended arms forward, hands down on the floor. His elbows are then rigidly extended, the arms adducted and internally rotated, hands fisted. Still later, he may get about on his knees and "bunny hop" on his fully flexed legs. A few children can even raise their trunks and hop on their knees without arm support.

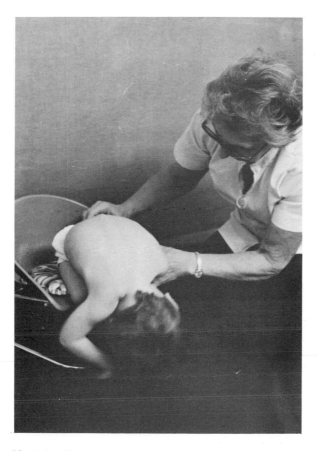

Fig. 39a Athetoid quadruplegia. Sitting: Total collapse in flexion when hips are flexed.

The athetoid child usually does not creep in prone or crawl reciprocally on hands and knees. Some children, whose legs can adduct, will learn to sit on the floor even without supporting themselves with their arms. They maintain the sitting position and balance with strong hip flexion and, as they can move their legs well, they may even get about on their seats (Figs 44a, b). However, although sitting fairly

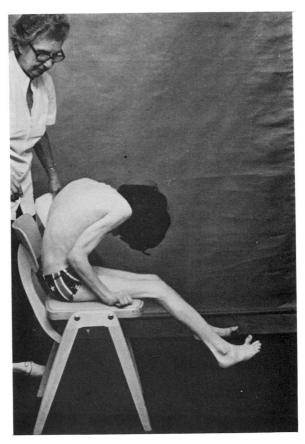

Fig. 39b Athetoid quadruplegia. Sitting: Excessive flexion of trunk when hips are flexed.

safely on the floor, they may not be able to sit and balance on a chair or stool without support (Fig. 45). The reason for this is that flexion of the knees, added to that of the hips, results in a total flexor pattern of the whole body.

When well supported in a chair with a table in front, the child feels safe and tries to use his hands, but usually can use only one hand at a time, often only the left one (Fig. 46). The

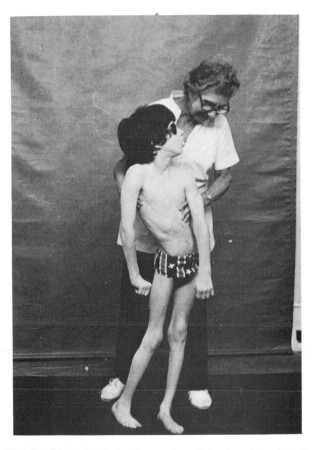

Fig. 40 Athetoid quadruplegia. Asymmetry of trunk and head posture producing scoliosis of spine.

only way his hands can meet in midline is with flexion forward of head and spine. His elbows are then also flexed, arms adducted and hands fisted (Fig. 47). If he extends his head and spine, he may be able to lift one arm with a rigidly extended elbow, and, by bending his wrist, his hand may open (Fig. 48). In this way, he may learn to type with one finger.

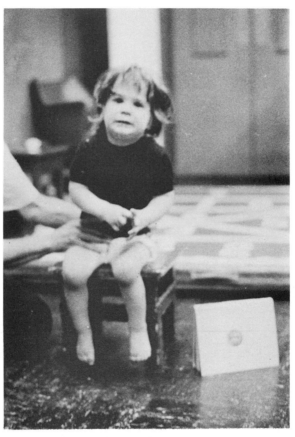

Fig. 41 Athetoid quadruplegia. Sitting: Lack of arm support, no balance of trunk.

The grasp of the athetoid hand is weak and unsustained. His hand, at rest, is usually open, with some flexion at wrist and elbow. The athetoid child withdraws his hand instead of grasping when approached by the examiner's hand or when he is being presented with an object. Twitchell (1959) has

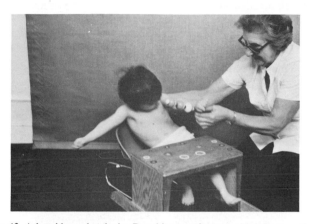

Fig. 42 Athetoid quadruplegia. Reaching out for toy with left arm, elbow rigidly extended and hand fisted, right arm pulling backwards extended. Note: Extension of left leg, hips and trunk.

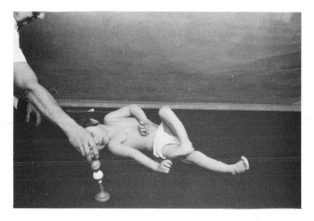

Fig. 43 Athetoid quadruplegia. Rolling initiated with leg, shoulder follows.

described this difficulty of grasping and has called it "avoidance reaction". If the child should succeed in grasping the object, he soon drops it again.

Independent movements of the eyes, that is, independent from movements of the head, are difficult or impossible for most children with athetoid quadruplegia. This means that, if they want to look at an object or a person, they have to move

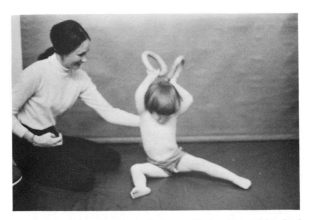

Fig. 44a Athetoid quadruplegia. Sitting and balancing with hip flexion.

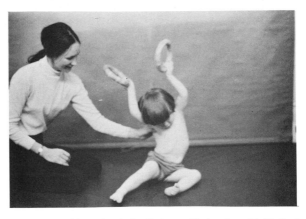

Fig. 44b Athetoid quadruplegia. Sitting and balancing with hip flexion.

the head. As they lack trunk stability and balance, any movement of the head affects the whole body and limbs. This makes independent use of arms and hands impossible and interferes with eye-hand co-ordination. Looking upwards, without thrusting the head and trunk backwards, is often a great problem. As the head is usually turned to one preferred side, looking to the opposite side is also difficult for many

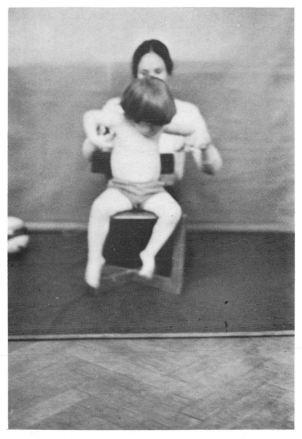

Fig. 45 Athetoid quadruplegia. Though sitting safely on the floor, no balance sitting on chair.

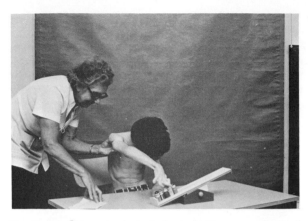

Fig. 46 Athetoid quadruplegia. In front of table can use one hand.

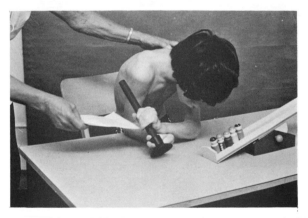

Fig. 47 Athetoid quadruplegia. Use of both hands with excessive flexion of body.

children. In a few children there is nystagmus, but even if there is none, focusing for any length of time, or scanning a line, is difficult or impossible, a fact which makes reading very difficult. Another problem is that they cannot look at the hand they are using but turn the head away from it (Fig. 49).

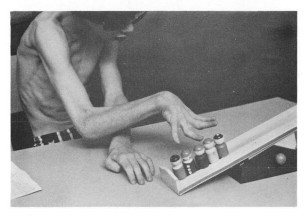

Fig. 48 Athetoid quadruplegia. His hand opens by bending his wrist.

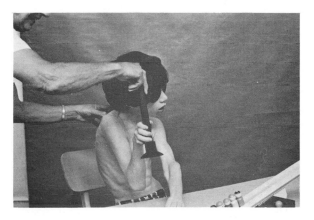

Fig. 49 Athetoid quadruplegia. Looking to the opposite side of the hand he uses.

Third stage. Standing and walking

Standing is achieved very late, even in children who are intelligent, and whose legs are less affected than their trunks and upper limbs. Many athetoid children do not get on to their feet at all and, as they sit most of the time, in a wheelchair, or well supported on a chair, with a table in front, they may develop flexor deformities at hips and knees. Standing is only possible if the legs are fairly normal and if they can extend their hips and knees with abducted legs. The greatest difficulty for standing up is their inability to use their hands for pulling themselves up to standing by holding onto a support. The extension they need for upright standing makes them thrust head and trunk backwards, together with

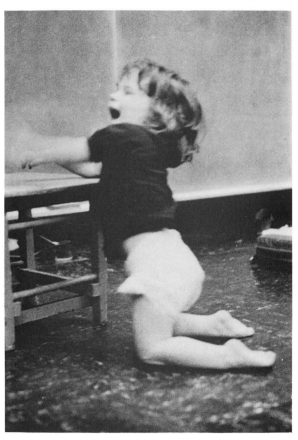

Fig. 50a Athetoid quadruplegia. Kneeling to stand up. Note: Wide opening of mouth with effort of extension.

retraction of the arms at the shoulders. A few children stand up by getting onto their knees first, then putting their flexed arms onto a chair and pulling themselves up on to their feet (Figs 50a, b, c). They then raise the head and extend the hips by pushing the pelvis forward. With this extension, the shoulders retract, both arms being flexed at the elbows or, if the head is turned to one side, one arm is flexed, the other extended. The children hyper-extend their knees for stability,

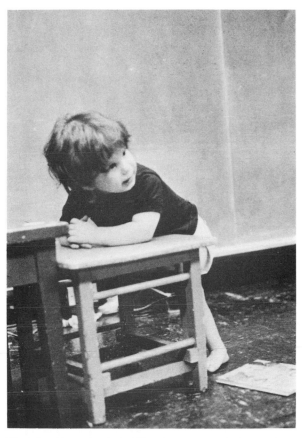

Fig. 50b Athetoid quadruplegia. Flexed arm on chair for pulling herself up.

as the slightest degree of flexion at hips or knees will lead to a collapse in flexion. There is a tendency for one leg only to take weight while the other pulls up in flexion or "paws" the ground with alternate flexion and extension. The child may learn to make voluntary use of the asymmetrical tonic neck reflex by turning his head towards that side in order to help extension and weight-bearing on the "flexor leg" (Fig. 51).

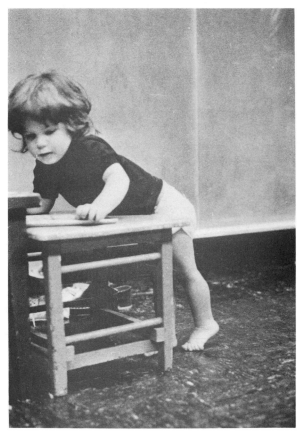

Fig. 50c Athetoid quadruplegia. Stands and plays with arm support on chair. Note: "Clawing" of toes of left foot.

Standing balance is difficult and is only achieved after a very long time. Shoulder and neck retraction help the child to stand up against gravity but they also make him lean backwards with his trunk. Therefore, in order to prevent

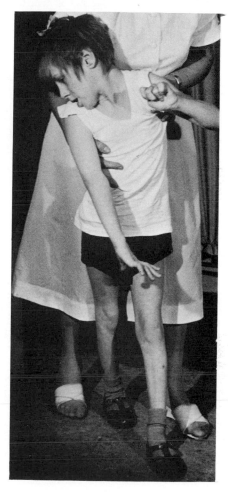

Fig. 51 Athetoid quadruplegia. Use of asymmetrical tonic neck reflex to help weight-bearing on right leg.

himself from falling backwards, he either pushes his head and chin forward, or he presses his chin down onto his chest (Figs 52a, b). This flexion of the head makes it possible for him to move his arms forward and down with extended elbows and to hold his hands together in front. In this way, he manages to stabilise shoulder-girdle and trunk, while the pushing forward of his pelvis, with extension of the hips, provides sufficient extension of the legs for weight-bearing.

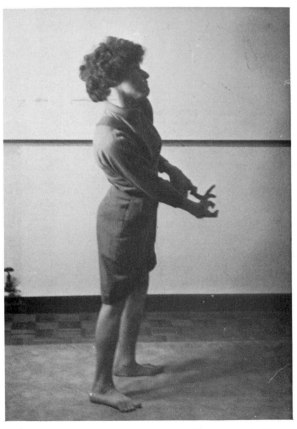

Fig. 52a Athetoid quadruplegia. Pushing chin forward and holding hands together against falling backwards.

Walking unaided is also very late and only those children who are moderately or slightly affected get to this stage. We have seen patients who did not achieve it until 15 years of age. When they attempt to take their first steps unaided, they tend to collapse due to sudden flexor spasms. At first, they often lift their feet too high which makes them lose their balance. They gradually learn to avoid the flexion which makes them collapse and to keep their hips and knees

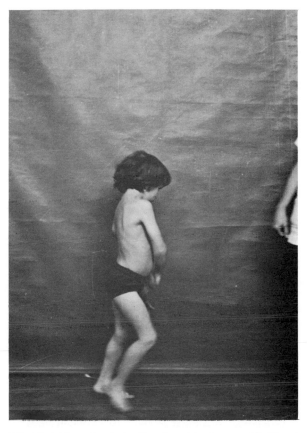

Fig. 52b Athetoid quadruplegia. Pressing chin down and holding hands together against falling backwards.

somewhat extended, "shuffling" along without lifting their legs or putting one foot in front of the other. The weight is on the medial border of their feet, with resulting valgus deformities.

A few children, who are only slightly affected, may learn to walk on a smaller base, putting one foot in front of the other. Their gait is unsteady, jerky and very asymmetrical. One leg leads, the other follows, without really stepping forward in front of the other. They are usually able to maintain balance by taking steps backwards, when in danger of falling back. Standing is more difficult than walking and they are unable to stand still for any length of time because of the need to take steps backward in order to balance.

SPASTIC QUADRUPLEGIA

1 The severely affected children

In these children, the prognosis is bad, even when they are treated early in life, as spasticity or rigidity is already strong at a few weeks or months of age. Epilepsy may be present early or develop later on. Fits may be of all kinds: myoclonic jerks, petit mal, or major convulsions. Microcephaly and various degrees of mental subnormality may be associated with a child's physical handicap. In some children, there are visual defects, partial or total blindness, or visual agnosia. Hearing defects or auditory imperception may also be present.

In supine, opisthotonous, together with a complete lack of head control, are early symptoms, as are a rigidly extended spine with shoulder retraction, adductor spasticity and excessive extension of the legs. Contractures of the adductors may develop very early on and be equally strong, with flexed or extended legs. In the early stages, there may not yet be internal rotation of the legs at the hips but this will develop later on. To begin with, the ankles may still be dorsiflexed, but they will soon plantiflex, when the child is left lying on his back for most of the day, or when he is put on his feet to try to make him stand. Asymmetrical tonic neck reflexes are usually pronounced, the head preferably turned to one side with lateral flexion of the neck to the opposite side. There may be resistance to turning the child's face to the opposite side. The lateral flexion of the neck will affect the whole spine, resulting in asymmetry of the trunk and obliquity of the pelvis. This is associated with a dysplasia of the hip and often with a subluxation or dislocation of, usually, the left hip (Fig. 53). In some cases, adductor

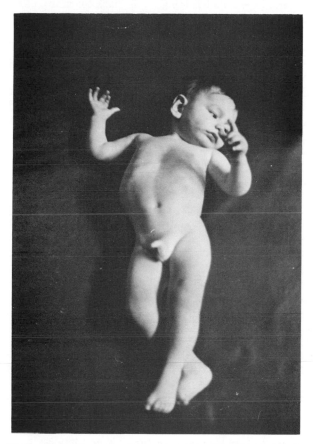

Fig. 53 Spastic quadruplegia. Asymmetry of trunk with lateral flexion of neck, obliquity of pelvis, internal rotation and adduction of left leg. Note: External rotation and flexion of right leg.

spasticity and internal rotation of the legs may produce dislocation of both hips.

When placed in prone-lying, the child cannot lift his head and extend his spine and hips. He may not even be able to turn his head to one side to free his airways, and he will dislike prone-lying because of the difficulty of breathing in this position. His mother, therefore, will not put him into prone and he will be left lying on his back for many months.

He cannot sit unsupported and falls over to one side. His back is very round, his hips are insufficiently flexed and his legs are too much adducted to give him a sitting base. This, combined with the asymmetry of his spine, may produce a kyphoscoliosis.

Early, and for a long time to come, there are great feeding problems. Tongue-thrusts are frequent as well as difficulties of suckling and swallowing and the child may tend to choke when fed. Some children suffer from reversed breathing, or stridor and respiration present problems, especially at night.

Even early treatment may have only limited results in furthering the child's development. However, it can help to prevent some, if not most, of the contractures and deformities, which quickly develop, often in a matter of months. Treatment and advice on home management, especially in the early stages, when we do not yet know what potential the baby may have, are necessary to help and support the family. It helps the mother in handling the child with greater ease and more confidence.

2. The quadruplegic child who is less severely affected

Fortunately, the majority of spastic quadruplegias are not so severely affected as those described above. The milder cases develop spasticity more gradually during the first year of life, although early signs can often be detected at 3–4 months of age, sometimes even earlier. Spasticity may not become strong enough to prevent the child from moving. The distribution of spasticity always affects one side more than the other. It may be severe on one side and moderate on the other. It may be moderate on one side and slight on the other. This asymmetrical distribution of spasticity, as well as the exclusive use of one arm and hand only, favours a tendency to scoliosis. Whereas the severely involved child, who cannot move at all, becomes deformed by remaining in a few abnormal postures, the less severely affected child tries to move and function, but can do so only in a few abnormal ways, i.e. in stereotyped abnormal patterns and with excessive effort, which increases his spasticity. Sometimes children who have been diagnosed as spastic quadruplegias at 8 or 10 months of age develop athetoid movements later on, in addition to their spasticity. This usually happens when they become more active around 18 months to 2 years of age.

First stage. Supine, prone, sitting supported

The child is a very late developer. The first signs are lack of head control when pulled to sitting and the inability to lift the head in prone-lying (Fig. 54). He remains on his back and cannot roll over, not even to one side, and he cannot sit up.

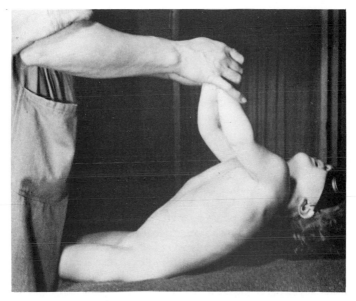

Fig. 54 Spastic quadruplegia. Lack of head control pulled to sitting.

When the child lies on his back, he holds his legs somewhat abducted and flexed, much like a normal baby of 2 or 3 months of age (Fig. 55). However, he hardly moves his legs and kicking is weak; usually the right leg moves more than the left and abducts with flexion. This asymmetrical

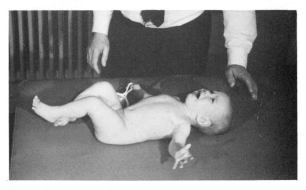

Fig. 55 Spastic quadruplegia. Legs show some abduction with flexion, right leg more flexed and abducted than left.

kicking of one leg tends to rotate the child's pelvis backwards on the right side which, in turn, produces adduction and internal rotation of the left leg. This pattern has to be watched carefully, as it is the forerunner of future subluxation or dislocation of the left hip. Kicking is usually confined to one or the other leg. The hips and knees remain in some flexion during the extensor phase. With semi-extension, we see some adduction and often, already at an early stage, internal rotation of the legs. Reciprocal kicking is rare and simultaneous kicking of both legs, normal at 4 or 5 months, does not develop at all. Neither do we find extension of the legs with abduction and external rotation, which a normal baby develops from 5 to 6 months onwards. The pattern of extension with abduction is a very important one in preparation for balance in standing and walking later on. Like the diplegic and hemiplegic children, the quadruplegic dorsiflexes his ankles only when bending hip and knee and he plantiflexes and supinates his feet when extending his legs.

The normal baby moves his ankles and toes independently of the position at hips and knees at a few weeks of age. The toes of the spastic child remain plantiflexed in a "grasp" position, a pattern similar to the fisting of his hands. It is interesting that, at this early stage, that is, before the child is made to stand or sit, his legs do not show much extensor or adductor spasticity (Fig. 56). Passive abduction with flexed legs may not be resisted although full abduction with extended legs may not be as easily obtained as in the normal baby. There is usually more resistance to abduction of the left leg than of the right.

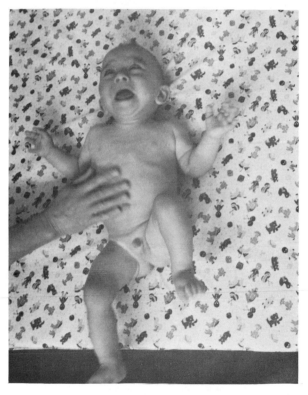

Fig. 56 Spastic quadruplegia. Flexion and abduction of legs early on.

In supine, there is strong retraction of the child's arms at the shoulder, with flexion of the elbows and fisted hands. He cannot reach forward and may only extend one arm when asymmetrical tonic neck reflexes act on the "face" arm (Fig. 57). The Moro reaction is maintained for a very long time, sometimes for years (Fig. 58). Asymmetrical tonic neck reflexes are present to both sides but often stronger to the

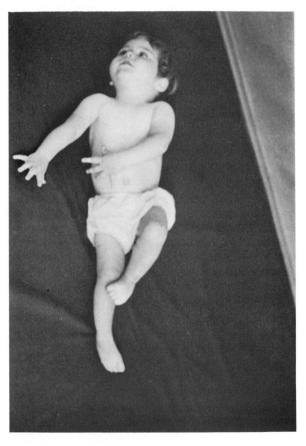

Fig. 57 Spastic quadruplegia. Asymmetrical tonic neck reflex with extension of the "face" arm and leg.

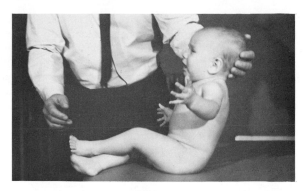

Fig. 58 Spastic quadruplegia. Moro reaction.

right, with the neck laterally flexed to the left. This, together with retraction of the shoulder-girdle, prevents the baby from getting his hands to his mouth and from engaging his hands in midline. Therefore he misses the normal symmetrical stage of trunk development, the bilateral use of his hands and the ability to transfer objects from one hand to the other. He cannot reach out for and grasp objects or put them to his mouth, as normal babies do.

In prone-lying, his trunk is flexed and his shoulders protracted (Fig. 59). His arms are adducted and often caught underneath his chest. There is also flexion of hips and knees

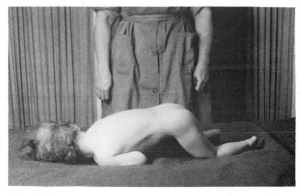

Fig. 59 Spastic quadruplegia. Total flexor pattern in prone-lying.

and passive extension may be strongly resisted. The child cannot lift his head, though he may be able to turn his face to one side, but, usually not to the other. He cannot move his arms out from under his chest or forward to support himself on his forearms. Therefore, he is uncomfortable and objects to being put into prone-lying and cries. When his head is passively lifted, there is strong resistance of neck and trunk and he cannot use his arms for support; they pull up in flexion so that he "hangs by the neck". Head-raising may be helped by extending his hips, but then his legs adduct and extend stiffly (Fig. 60). The normal child initiates extension of

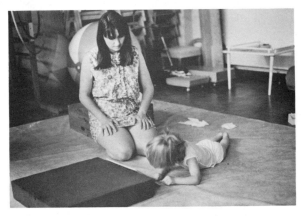

Fig. 60 Spastic quadruplegia. Head raising with adducted stiffly extended legs.

the spine and hips by lifting his head first and by supporting himself on his forearms. In contrast to the spastic child, the normal baby's legs remain abducted and flexed and they remain abducted when they extend, i.e. at about 5–6 months of age. At this stage, the normal baby can also push himself up on his extended arms, which the spastic quadruplegic child cannot do.

When sitting supported, the quadruplegic child's back is very round. Like the diplegic child, he sits on his sacrum and has to bring his trunk forward over the sitting base with a compensatory kyphosis. His head falls forward and down

(Fig. 61). As the posture of his trunk is asymmetrical, with lateral flexion of his neck, this adds a scoliosis to the kyphosis. Initially, the spine is mobile and can be straightened out by bringing the head into midline. It indicates, however, a possible future permanent kypho-scoliosis. The child's legs are now adducted and semiflexed with plantiflexion of the ankles and toes (Fig. 62). In spite of the flexion of spine and neck, the arms retract at the shoulders, the elbows are flexed and pronated and the hands fisted. In this position of flexion, he can only look downwards. In order to give the child a chance to see people and his surroundings, he is supported in half-lying. When he sits on his mother's lap, he leans backwards and also tends to push himself backwards. His hips and legs then extend, adduct and often cross.

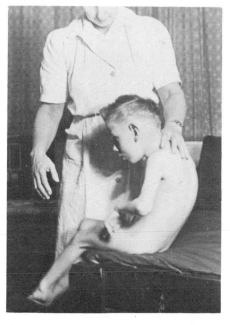

Fig. 61 Spastic quadruplegia. Sitting on sacrum, kyphosis, and head down.

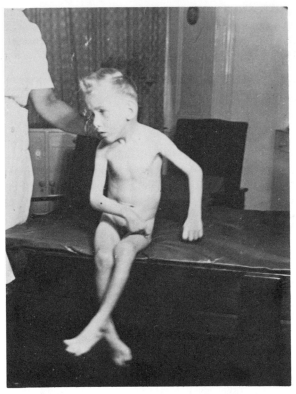

Fig. 62 Spastic quadruplegia. Sitting, legs adducted with plantiflexion of ankles and toes.

Second stage. Sitting and rolling over

Gradually, the child develops some head control in sitting and counteracts falling backwards by voluntary flexion of his head. When pulled to sitting, he still has an initial head lag and rights his head only when his hips are in some flexion, that is, about half-way up to sitting. He cannot lift his head from supine and he cannot reach forward and extend his arms to grasp his mother's hands to assist being pulled to sitting. In sitting, his arms may now protract at the shoulders as part of the voluntary flexion of head and trunk, instead of the former retraction, and his arms are stiff in flexion and pronation. Due to having been made to sit supported for a great length of time, flexor hypertonus becomes so strong that some children can even lift the head from supine, though they are unable to do so from prone-lying. Having achieved some head control in sitting, the child can now look forwards but if he looks upwards, he will still tend to fall back if unsupported, and, if supported, to push himself backwards. A startle reaction or even a Moro reaction may persist for many years in spite of some head control forwards. In some children, however, the flexor pattern and flexor spasticity may become so strong that these reactions are inhibited and cannot occur. This excessive flexion will then interfere with the development of arm support with extended arms (the parachute reaction) and also with the ability to reach forward and upward with the hands.

Contractures of the flexors and pronators of the elbows develop gradually in many children. A few children may learn to use one arm and hand sideways for support, or one hand for crude grasp and release of objects. Though a child can control the head to some extent in sitting, he cannot move it independently from the trunk and he does not develop trunk balance. Every movement of his head sideways or backwards makes him fall over unless his trunk is supported (Figs 63a, b).

The quadruplegic child spends most of his day in supported sitting, or strapped to a chair. His legs are adducted and flexed at hips and knees and he is thus prevented from learning to balance at the hips or to develop his own active trunk control. He learns to feed himself without being able to lift his arms to get his hands to his mouth and therefore has to bend his head down to his hand, increasing the flexion of hips and knees and the danger of developing flexor contractures. He uses the same pattern of flexion for grasping and manipulation of objects and when learning to write.

Though supported sitting may have improved and a child be able to use at least one hand to some extent, for many children rolling over from supine to prone is still difficult or impossible. They may be able to roll over to one side only,

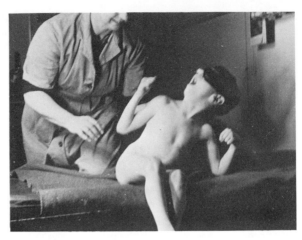

Fig. 63a Spastic quadruplegia. Movement of the head sideways makes child fall to that side.

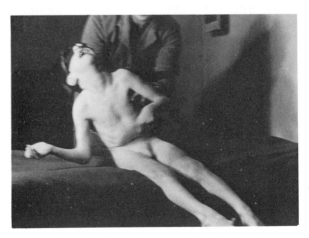

Fig. 63b Spastic quadruplegia. Movement of head backwards makes child fall back.

using the less affected side to do so. They use a total flexor pattern of the whole body to do this, without rotation of the spine and without extension of the hips (Fig. 64). Only those

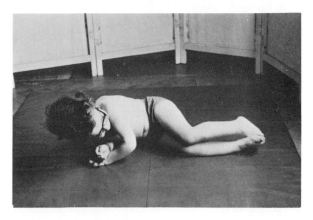

Fig. 64 Spastic quadruplegia. Rolling over in total flexor pattern.

children who can lift the head in prone-lying can turn over completely to prone. However, as at best they can raise themselves up on to their forearms but cannot extend one arm to reach out for a toy, they are unable to use their hands in prone-lying. They therefore dislike this position and would rather remain on their backs when put on the floor.

Third stage. Progression on the floor, sitting unsupported, standing and walking

Only those children with moderate spasticity will reach this stage. When prone on the floor, they get about much like the diplegic children and pull themselves forward with flexed and pronated arms and fisted hands, dragging their stiffly extended adducted legs behind them. Whereas the diplegic child can push himself backwards with his arms onto his knees when trying to get up, the quadruplegic child puts his head down and, with full flexion of trunk and arms, pulls his knees under his abdomen (Figs 65a, b). He then sits back on his feet but he may not be able to extend his arms to raise his body. He will remain on his forearms and only lift his head to look around. Some children are able to lift the head, extend the arms somewhat and raise the trunk. They then sit back between the feet, like the diplegic children (Figs 66a, b, c).

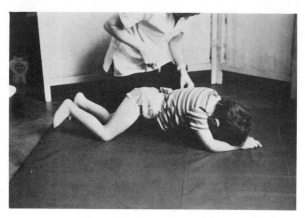

Fig. 65a Spastic quadruplegia. Child puts his head down and pulls his knees under his abdomen using flexor patterns to get on to his knees.

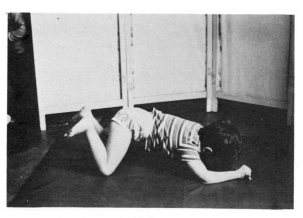

Fig. 65b Spastic quadruplegia. Child puts his head down and pulls his knees under his abdomen, using flexor pattern to get on to his knees. Note: He cannot push himself up with his arms.

Getting about on hands and knees is very difficult and slow, as the arms are too stiff in semi-flexion. This means that the children spend their days kneeling, crawling or sitting. They cannot yet stand and they no longer like prone-lying on the floor, an activity which gave them some extension earlier on

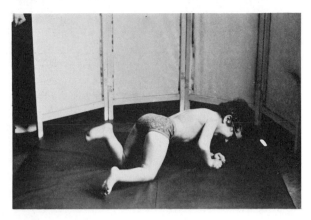

Fig. 66a Spastic quadruplegia. Child can lift his head and get on to his semi-flexed arms.

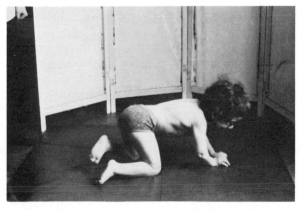

Fig. 66b Spastic quadruplegia. Child raises his trunk and gets on hands and knees.

when they pulled themselves along the floor instead of crawling on all fours, which they now prefer. All their activities are now done with too much flexion of trunk and limbs and thus flexor spasticity increases still further. This results in contractures and deformities in flexion of spine, hips and knees.

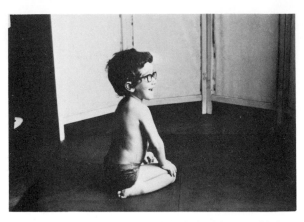

Fig. 66c Spastic quadruplegia. Child sits back between his feet.

Only slightly affected spastic quadruplegias, or those who are slightly affected on one side and moderately on the other, may attain sitting unsupported with trunk balance, and then progress to standing up. In order to achieve this, they need at least one arm which is good enough for reaching out and for grasping and holding onto a support. This enables them to pull themselves up to standing or to sit up from lying on their backs. They cannot get up to sitting from prone-lying, however, because they would need arm support and, especially, rotation of the trunk. Normal babies do this at about 8 months, long before they push themselves up to sitting from supine.

Walking unaided, even abnormally, is impossible for most of these children because of the balance problems and the very narrow standing base. They stand on their toes with stiffly extended, or semi-flexed, adducted and internally rotated legs (Fig. 67).

Conclusion The motor development of the child with cerebral palsy shows some typical features which have been described in this book. The child's postural tone and his motor patterns change as he grows and develops. Cerebral palsy is not easy to diagnose in the very young child, unless he is severely affected. Spasticity or athetosis is slight, or

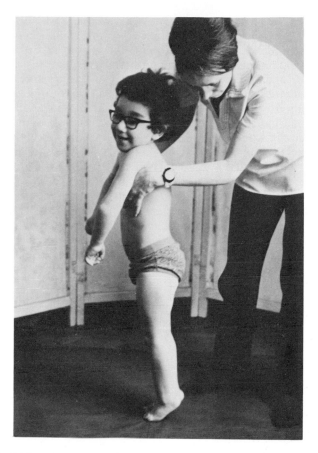

Fig. 67 Spastic quadruplegia. Standing on his toes with adducted legs. Note: Internal rotation of arms and legs.

even absent, at first, and no deformities are present. The picture changes throughout the years.

The described sequences of abnormal development in different types of cerebral palsy have been observed on a great number of children, many of whom had already spontaneously developed their abnormal activities before attending for treatment. It is important to know the sequences of abnormal motor development in order to anticipate their occurrence in very young children. It also helps to detect the first signs of abnormal postural behaviour and to recognise its implication for the future activities of the child and the possible development of contractures and deformities. In the older child, it enables one to look both backwards and forwards — that is, to understand what has caused the child's present problems as well as to anticipate what might happen in the future. This knowledge will help to plan treatment with a view to preventing abnormality instead of trying to correct it afterwards, as well as avoiding further deterioration. Though a child with cerebral palsy cannot develop normally or go through all the stages of normal child development, carefully planned treatment and home management can and should help to counteract the abnormal patterns of posture and movement at their earliest signs. At the same time, the child can be given the most essential preparatory movement patterns necessary for the activities he is trying to perform, or should require at his age and stage of development. Treatment has been described in former papers (Bobath, K. and B., 1963, 1964, 1967, 1971) and home management by Finnie, N. (1968).

APPENDIX

Some Aspects of Development for Comparison and Diagnosis

	The normal child	*The cerebral palsied child*
a) **First three months**	A great variety of movements. Independent movements of knees, ankles and toes. Firm grasp.	Stereotyped few movements. Total patterns of flexion and extension. No grasp.
b) **Four months**	*Head control and symmetry* Head steady when child moved. Midline orientation, hands together, to mouth, to clothes.	Lack of head control. Head turned to one side. Uses only one hand, hands do not engage.
c) **Five to six months**	*Extension — abduction of arms and legs* Landau begins, stands supported, legs adducted, external rotation. Reaches out with arms forward.	No Landau, adduction with internal rotation of legs, retraction of shoulders. No reach forward with arms.
d) **Six to seven months**	Arm support forwards and sideways. Pulls to sit up. Lifts head from supine. Prone on extended arms. Rolls prone to supine. Moro gone.	No arm support, sitting or prone. Does not pull to sit. Cannot lift head from supine. Cannot roll, no rotation. Moro may continue.
e) **Seven to eight months**	*Sitting and sitting up from prone unaided* Creeps on abdomen, pivots sitting, pulls himself to stand.	Sitting falls over sideways or backwards. Cannot sit up from prone. Cannot creep on abdomen.
f) **Nine to ten months**	*Standing legs wide apart* Stands holding on to furniture, lifts one foot. Walks along furniture. Crawls on hands and knees. Landau strong.	Stood up, legs adducted. Does not pull himself to stand. No Landau.

BIBLIOGRAPHY

Bobath, B. Treatment principles and planning in cerebral palsy. *Physiotherapy,* April 1963.

A neuro-developmental treatment of cerebral palsy. *Physiotherapy,* August 1963.

The very early treatment of cerebral palsy. *Developmental Medicine and Child Neurology,* Vol. 9, No. 4, August 1967, pp. 373–390.

Motor development, its effect on general development and application to the treatment of cerebral palsy. *Physiotherapy,* November 1971.

Bobath, K. The normal postural reflex mechanism and its deviation in children with cerebral palsy. *Physiotherapy,* November 1971.

Bobath, K. and Bobath, B. The facilitation of normal postural reactions in the treatment of cerebral palsy. *Physiotherapy,* August 1964.

The neurodevelopmental treatment of cerebral palsy. *Journal of the American Physical Therapy Association,* Vol. 47, 1967.

André-Thomas, Yves Chesni and St. Anne Dargassies. The neurological examination of the infant. *Little Club Clinics in Developmental Medicine,* No. 1, 1960, pp. 29–31.

Doran Benyon, Sheila. *Intensive Programming for Slow Learners.* Charles E. Merrill Publishing Co., Columbus, Ohio, pp. 11–24.

Finnie, N. *Handling the Young Cerebral Palsied Child at Home.* William Heinemann Medical Books Ltd. Second Edition. 1974.

Illingworth, R. S. *The Development of the Infant and the Young Child, Normal and Abnormal.* E. & S. Livingstone, Edinburgh and London, 1960, p. 140.

Ingram, T. T. S. Muscle tonus and posture in infancy. *Cerebral Palsy Bulletin,* No. 5, pp. 6 and 31.

MacKeith, R. The primary walking response and its facilitation by passive extension of the head. *Escratti da "Acta Paed. Latina",* Vol. XVII. Supplied as Rasc. 6, 1964.

Milani-Comparetti, A. Spasticity versus patterned postural and motor behaviour of spastics. From *Excerpta Medica International Congress Series, No. 107, Proceedings of the IVth International Congress of Physical Medicine,* Paris 6–11th September 1964.

Robson, P. Variations of normal motor development. *Study Group on Promoting Better Movement in Children with Motor Handicap.* Nottingham, September 1973.

Shuffling, hitching, scooting or sliding. *Developmental Medicine and Child Neurology.* October 1970, No. 5, pp. 608–617.

Rosenberg, B. and Weller, G. M. Minor physical anomalies and academic performance in young school children. *Developmental Medicine and Child Neurology,* 1973, No. 15, pp. 131–135.

Twitchell, T. E. On the motor deficit in congenital bilateral athetosis. *Journal of Nervous and Mental Diseases,* Vol. 129, No. 2, August 1959.

INDEX

104